T0296134

FAST FACTS FOR THE TRAVEL NURSE

Travel Nursing in a Nutshell

About the Author

Michele Angell Landrum, RN, received her Associate Degree in Nursing from the University of Mobile in 1998. She worked as a travel nurse for eight years in various locations throughout the United States. Her specialties include the open-heart recovery unit, the intensive care unit, the emergency room, the cardiac catheterization lab, the electro physiology lab, and the special procedures lab.

She is currently employed by Cardiology Associates in Mobile, Alabama, where she works in the CT department, and by Springhill Medical Center, also located in Mobile, where she is a clinical nurse educator with the staff development department.

FAST FACTS FOR THE TRAVEL NURSE

Travel Nursing in a Nutshell

Michele Angell Landrum, RN

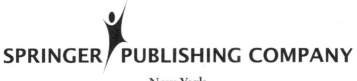

SPRINGER PUBLISHING COMPANY

New York

Springer Publishing Company, LLC
11 West 42nd Street
New York, NY 10036
www.springerpub.com

Acquisitions Editor: Margaret Zuccarini
Project Manager: Barbara Chernow
Cover Design: David Levy
Composition: Agnew's, Inc.

E-book ISBN: 978-0-8261-3787-6

10 11 12/ 5 4 3 2 1

The author and the publisher of this Work have made every effort to use sources believed to be reliable to provide information that is accurate and compatible with the standards generally accepted at the time of publication. Because medical science is continually advancing, our knowledge base continues to expand. Therefore, as new information becomes available, changes in procedures become necessary. We recommend that the reader always consult current research and specific institutional policies before performing any clinical procedure. The author and publisher shall not be liable for any special, consequential, or exemplary damages resulting, in whole or in part, from the readers' use of, or reliance on, the information contained in this book. The publisher has no responsibility for the persistence or accuracy of URLs for external or third-party Internet Web sites referred to in this publication and does not guarantee that any content on such Web sites is, or will remain, accurate or appropriate.

Library of Congress Cataloging-in-Publication Data

Landrum, Michele Angell.
  Fast facts for the travel nurse : travel nursing in a nutshell / Michele Angell Landrum.
    p. ; cm.
  Includes bibliographical references and index.
  ISBN 978-0-8261-3786-9
  1. Travel nursing. I. Title.
  [DNLM 1. Nursing—United States. 2. Travel—United States. 3. Vocational
Guidance—United States. WY 101 L262f 2010]
  RT120.T73L36 2010
  616.9'802—dc22
                                                                2009042088

Printed in the United States of America by Hamilton Printing Company.

This book is dedicated to my husband, Ted, for his love, friendship, encouragement, strength, and support during the writing of this guide, as well as throughout our lives and careers. Without him, none of this would have been possible. And, to my amazing son, Carter, I have been blessed by your love and have found strength in being your mother.

—MAL

Contents

Preface

Would you like to learn how to make your job the adventure of a lifetime and finance your dreams at the same time? If so, this book is the guide that will help you navigate the travel nursing trail and achieve that goal. First, you should understand why travel nurses are in high demand. Second, you need to discover what makes a travel-nursing career so appealing—and, here, the reasons are so numerous that discussing them all is impossible.

The primary reason for the high demand is the nursing shortage in the United States. As of 2007, the American Hospital Association reported that the number of vacant nursing positions was 116,000. In March 2008, Dr. Peter Buerhaus and his colleagues reported that this figure is expected to increase to 500,000 by 2025.*

These numbers guarantee the continued employment of registered nurses and fuel the fire of the travel nursing industry. The reasons for this shortage range from the retirement of current practicing RNs to fewer nurse educators to a lower

*The Future of the Nursing Workforce in the United States: Data, Trends and Implications, Sudbury, MA: Jones and Bartlett.

number of students enrolling in nursing programs. Add to this mix the aging U.S. population, and a fantastic opportunity is just waiting for you to grab hold.

This prospect offers both a good income and exciting experiences, which provide sufficient reason for you to entertain the idea of a travel assignment. The flexibility of lifestyle and schedule is a great perk, and the friends you will make along the way are an invaluable benefit. But one of the greatest advantages of being a travel nurse is job satisfaction.

Job satisfaction is very high among travelers because they are in control of their location, facility, and unit each and every 13 weeks. A traveler has the ability to change one, or all, of these variables with each new contract. The pay is amazing, and you will be learning constantly while on the job and at "home." All of these features make for an extraordinary career.

We all entered the nursing field to help others. We follow in the path of Florence Nightingale, the original "nurse," who fought for safer and more effective ways to help and heal patients. As we move through our nursing careers, many of us start to lose that feeling. We become overworked and underappreciated. Job satisfaction slips lower and lower, until sometimes, a nurse will consider leaving the field all together.

Travel nursing offers a great escape from this dissatisfaction. You will go to a facility that knows it needs you, and your pay will, in most cases, increase substantially. In addition, each new location and facility will provide a change of pace that provides a new adventure. If the idea of travel nursing scares you, try it for a short time. Take a leave of absence from your current position and try a four-, six-, or eight-week assignment. No loss; no long-term commitment.

For me, working as a travel nurse renewed my sense of purpose. I became excited about nursing again. This feeling deepened with each new assignment and locale. I have learned so many things, professionally and personally, that have made me so thankful for this fantastic opportunity.

Even Dear Abbey has expressed her opinion about the fabulous advantages of travel nursing. In an article posted in *The Daily Herald* of Everett, Washington, on August 30, 2006 (page E6), she addressed the issue of job dissatisfaction and disappointment among nurses. She urged her readers to consider a change in unit and/or location before leaving the field entirely. One option discussed was travel nursing. She suggested readers should consider all options before leaving the field of nursing and mentioned that with an alternative like travel nursing the reader might be "pleasantly surprised."

Dear Abby sure had it right. With all its advantages, travel nursing offers a great alternative to "regular" hospital nursing. This type of career offers exceptional compensation and a positive work environment, along with engaging patient care sets. The public knows that nurses are needed and working as a travel nurse is a well-respected part of the profession. With that said and all the positive benefits, what is there to lose? We have worked so hard for our licenses, education, and livelihood. Let's enjoy the work again, while reaping the rewards.

I was a travel nurse for eight years. My husband, a union electrician, and I went to terrific locations, such as New York, Los Angeles, San Francisco, Napa Valley, and Alaska. We had great experiences at locales throughout the state of Washington and spent ten absolutely amazing months in Hawaii! In addition, we explored other places on our way to these assignments.

This book is not designed as a technical manual. Rather, it contains useful information, easy to use checklists, and practical study guides. I wrote it for my friends, family members, and coworkers, who were always asking for my advice about how to get started and enjoy the traveling aspect of nursing. This is a one-to-one guide to help you plot a course through that world. By following these guidelines, you will make your job the adventure of a lifetime!

Good Luck!

Acknowledgments

Thank you to all the friends, fellow travelers, facility staff members, and staffing companies that made my travel-nurse career such a fantastic journey. Their help and guidance allowed me to grow personally, and professionally in ways I never imagined.

I would also like to recognize Margaret Zuccarini, Brian O'Connor, and Barbara Chernow for the invaluable insight, advice, and knowledge they so graciously shared with me. It allowed this manuscript to flourish.

A special thank you to Peggy Harris for her friendship, guidance, and support.

To my mother, Vera, thanks so much for your unwavering support, encouragement, and belief in my abilities. To my son, Carter, you were so patient and understanding while this manuscript was being developed and written. Without even knowing, you helped with every aspect of this book. Finally, to my husband Ted—you are my reference tool, editor, therapist, and, most importantly, my rock of strength. Thank you.

Part I

The Basics

All You'll Need to Know to Choose Your First Assignment

Chapter 1

Qualifications and Organization

INTRODUCTION

Choosing the right travel staffing company and finding your first travel assignment are two important factors in beginning a successful and satisfying travel-nursing career. The first step is to get organized. This chapter discusses the minimal qualifications necessary to become a travel nurse and provides the essentials for organizing the necessary paperwork to start your journey, as summarized in Exhibit 1.1 and Exhibit 1.2.

In this chapter, you will learn:

1. The general qualifications required to become a travel nurse.
2. The documents a prospective travel staffing company and the facilities to which you travel will require.
3. How to assemble a notebook that will allow you to access your paperwork with ease.

QUALIFICATIONS

All you need to qualify as a travel nurse is a current nursing license in good standing and one year of nursing experience. Any field of hospital nursing is acceptable. For example, you may be an emergency room (ER), intensive care unit (ICU), cardiac catheterization lab, telemetry, or operating room (OR) nurse. This is not to say that other fields of nursing do not have travel positions, but hospital nursing is usually the easiest arena in which to find travel assignments. Essentially, your RN license and the abovementioned experience is all you need. However, Exhibit 1.1 lists some additional requirements that might be needed for particular specialties.

Fast facts in a nutshell

One year of RN experience and a current nursing license is required to become a travel nurse.

EXHIBIT 1.1	Examples of Additional Certifications Required by Some Nursing Departments
Certification	Department
BLS	All nursing departments
ACLS	ER, ICU, CCU, Cardiac Cath Lab, etc.
PALS	ER, Pediatrics, PICU
NALS	Neonatal ICU
TNCC	Trauma ICU, Trauma ER

DOCUMENTATION

Travel staffing companies and the facilities at which you accept assignments will require several documents. **The key to managing all of this documentation is organization.** A large three-ring binder with tabs to separate your paperwork into specific groupings will make finding everything easy. Exhibit 1.2 lists the documents you will need before beginning your first travel assignment. The staffing companies will request this paperwork and will forward the information to prospective assignment facilities.

The laboratory work needed should remain the same for each company and facility. **Titers for your childhood immunizations will be required.** Rubeola, rubella, mumps, varicella zoster, and hepatitis-B will generally be all that are necessary. If you do not have current titers, the staffing company that you choose to take an assignment with will order them. The titers may be drawn by a local laboratory at the staffing company's expense. Verify that the laboratory used has authorization to perform the tests for your particular travel company before scheduling your appointment for the blood draw. **Be prepared to perform a urine drug screen the same day.**

A physical, completed by a physician, will be required. Most travel companies do not pay for this. If you do not have a copy of a documented physical in the last year, have one performed by the doctor of your choosing. No specific credentials are required for the physician completing the exam.

It is a good idea to **use a physical assessment or statement-of-health form from one of the travel companies** you have contacted. This form will be in the packets that the companies send you or should be available on-line from most of their Web sites. Generally, a staffing company and/or facility

---

**EXHIBIT 1.2   Documents Needed to Begin
an Assignment**

---

1. Copies of current driver's license, certifications (e.g., BLS, ACLS), RN license(s), and insurance card.
2. Recent lab work (titers, PPD).
3. Copies of immunizations, including hepatitis B series.
4. Documentation of a current physical by a physician.
5. Résumé.
6. List of all addresses within the last seven years for a background check
7. List of references and letters of recommendation.

---

will accept any completed physician physical assessment form, regardless of which company logo is on it. An example of the statement-of-health form can be found in Appendix A.

A résumé is an integral part of your documentation. One page of clear and precise information is all that is needed. The maximum length should be two pages. Do not list personal information, such as marital status, number of children, social security number, or desired income. Provide an easy-to-read education and work history, along with any certifications and/or credentials you possess (e.g., ACLS, IABP, CVVHD). Be sure to list the number of beds in each unit or floor where you have work. If you have experience in an OR, cardiac catheterization lab, electro physiology lab, and/or special procedures lab, note the number of rooms for each facility.

Fast facts in a nutshell

Multiple documents will need to be assembled prior to applying for a travel nurse position.

NOTEBOOK ASSEMBLY

Purchase a large three-ring binder in which to compile all your required documents. Make a tab for each document section and keep copies of all the paperwork filed properly inside. These tabs will help you keep information regarding your travel assignments handy and should include copies of licenses, laboratory work, proof of immunizations, documentation of a current physical, your résumé, addresses for a background check, and references.

After you have assembled these documents, you will want to create a few additional tabs inside the notebook. For example, add a section that includes a list of contacts, such as fellow travelers, local assignment staff, and nurse managers. A tab that contains a copy of your current contract and all previous contracts serves as a great reference tool. Be sure to keep a copy of the study guides and tests that the staffing companies and/or facilities provide to you in case such testing is required in the future. A few hospitals might even accept copies of tests and course completions, such as HIPPA and fire safety, from other facilities.

Keep your notebook up to date and properly organized. The information contained will be helpful and extremely useful.

Fast facts in a nutshell: summary

Travel nursing offers career opportunities, along with adventure and experiences visiting new places. As this chapter illustrates, experience in your chosen field, along with a few specific certifications, are all that you need to quality for a travel nurse position. Be sure to assemble all the necessary documents and keep them organized in a three-ring binder.

Chapter 2

Choosing a Travel Staffing Company

INTRODUCTION

Choosing the first travel assignment is both exciting and challenging. Many considerations need to be taken into account. Finding a travel staffing company to represent you to the hospitals and facilities is the next step needed to embark on a successful traveling career, and it is a major landmark in your journey. You can choose from more than a hundred travel nurse companies, ranging from small local agencies to huge international conglomerates. With all the choices, it is easy to feel intimidated.

Chapter 2 provides all the information you need to choose a staffing company that suits your needs and provides the proper amount of support. Exhibits 2.1 to 2.3 list questions you should ask of a potential travel company recruiter.

In this chapter, you will learn:

1. How to interview a recruiter from a travel staffing company.
2. How to obtain accurate information regarding benefits from the recruiter.

3. What types of questions a staffing company recruiter will ask you.
4. Tips for handling recruiter difficulties.

NARROWING THE FIELD

The best way to begin searching for a staffing company is to talk to as many travelers as possible. This includes current travelers, former travelers, and even future travelers who are just starting to plan their own journeys. Ask with which companies these professionals have found success and which have let them down. Just remember not to let the horror stories discourage you. Some people accentuate the bad and leave out the good. Taking a traveling assignment will be one of the most rewarding experiences of your life.

Fast facts in a nutshell

Ask other travelers about their experiences with travel staffing companies.

Do your own research on the Internet. A list of companies, with their telephone numbers and Web addresses, can be found in Appendix C. Select five companies that peak your interest. Contact them following these directions:

1. Find a quiet space where you will be uninterrupted and can ask the recruiter questions and take notes. This is called an

"interview" because that is exactly what you need to do: **interview the recruiter.**
2. Call the 1-800 number for the staffing company. Tell the operator that you are a registered nurse who would like to speak with a nursing recruiter regarding a possible assignment with the company.
3. **Ask the recruiter the questions regarding assignment pay, insurance, and housing options** that are shown in Exhibits 2.1 to 2.3. If you are connected to voice mail, leave a message with a contact number and a time that it is convenient for you to conduct the "interview."

Fast facts in a nutshell

The initial contact with a travel staffing company is easily completed via a 1-800 number.

THE INTERVIEW

Once you contact a travel staffing company recruiter, you will want to ask several questions to determine if this company is the right one for you. **Pay and insurance are the two biggest considerations when choosing a company.** Housing, location, and available assignments are also very important. These considerations make up the total package of a travel assignment.

The term, assignment, simply refers to a 4-, 8-, or 13-week contract in which a nurse works at a specific facility in a cer-

tain location as arranged by the staffing company. Occasionally a contract can last longer, as much as 6 months to 2 years.

The basic questions to first ask the nurse recruiter are given in Exhibit 2.1.

EXHIBIT 2.1   Questions to Ask a Recruiter Regarding Pay, Hours, and Additional Reimbursements

---

1. What is the average hourly pay? The recruiter probably won't give you a specific amount, but she or he can give you an "average" pay rate for a particular area.
2. Is this pay rate based on a 36-, 40-, or 48-hour work week? Some companies will offer a higher rate of pay for more mandatory hours per week.
3. What is the average number of hours worked per week, and is mandatory overtime required?
4. Do the assignments offer guaranteed pay for the weekly contracted hours? Ask specifically if you can be sent home early and still be paid for the contracted number of hours. This is not always the case, so be sure to clarify the policy with each and every assignment. Get the hours contracted, along with the guarantee, documented in your contract. On a contract extension, verify that the guaranteed pay is noted.
5. What is the average amount for on-call and callback pay?
6. Is there a completion bonus offered for an assignment with this company?
    A. How is it taxed?
    B. When is the bonus received? Verify the number of hours needed to receive the completion bonus with each

(continued)

contract, as it is generally dependent on the number of
hours worked not the number of weeks completed.

7. Does the company offer vacation time, vacation pay, or sick
pay? This is not customary, but some companies do have a
way to work it into their travel nurse program.

8. Is there a bonus if you refer another medical professional
to the company? If so, what are the restrictions and/or
specifications on receiving the bonus?

9. Does the company provide a travel allowance? If so, do they
have to book your arrival and departure travel or can you?

10. Do the assignments provide a car or a car allowance? A rental
car or car allowance is usually offered for those positions that
require call as part of the assignment.

11. Does this company provide for continuing education?

12. Will you be reimbursed for certifications required on specific
assignments?

13. Will the company reimburse you for licenses needed for
each state? Is there reimbursement for costs associated with
obtaining said license?

14. Is there a 401(k)?
    A. What is the maximum percentage for employee
    contributions?
    B. Up to what percentage does the employer match?
    C. When do you become vested?

**Insurance is the next area that you must cover with
the recruiter before choosing a travel staffing company.** Exhibit 2.2 indicates which questions need to be asked of each
company.

**The last major issue to discuss with a recruiter is how
housing is handled.** Exhibit 2.3 covers the types of questions
to ask regarding housing during a travel assignment.

EXHIBIT 2.2   Questions to Ask a Recruiter Regarding Insurance Coverage

---

1. Does insurance coverage start the first day of an assignment, or is there a 30/90-day waiting period?
2. Does the company cover 100% of the cost for the insurance?
3. Will it cover your spouse and/or child? If so, what will the cost be to add one or both of them?
4. Does the type of insurance, or the cost, change with each assignment?
5. How long will you have insurance coverage once your assignment is complete?
6. Is this a PPO or an HMO?
7. What are the copay and the deductible?
8. Is there prescription coverage? If so, what is the copay for medication?
9. Is there a short-term disability plan, and what are the fees?
10. Is there a long-term disability plan, and what are the fees?
11. Does the company offer life insurance, and what is the cost?

EXHIBIT 2.3   Questions to Ask a Recruiter Specific to Housing Offered by a Travel Staffing Company

---

1. Is a one-bedroom apartment provided for each assignment, or is shared housing the norm?
2. Does this company use hotels, or the like, to house its nurses?
3. Is the apartment furnished?
   A. Are dishes and linens provided?
   B. Are a washer and dryer provided?

(continued)

4. Can housing be upgraded? This is not common, but some companies may upgrade housing for extensions or serial assignments. Occasionally, a fee can be paid for this. Upgraded housing can include many things. It may mean private housing, a bigger apartment, or a washer and dryer in the apartment.
5. What is the average subsidy for an assignment? A subsidy is a stipend received for providing your own housing.

Fast facts in a nutshell

Interviewing the travel staffing recruiter is crucial to selecting the appropriate company to contract with.

OTHER CONSIDERATIONS

Several other important factors should be considered before choosing a company. **Find out how many facilities the company contracts with** and in which locations. **If considering an assignment abroad, confirm that this company handles international travel.** Inquire about the number of travel nurses the company employs and how many of those RNs are currently on assignment.

Ask the recruiter what shifts the company primarily offers. Sometimes, only a night shift will be available in certain locations at certain times of the year or with a particular company. **Be sure you are clear as to what is available at the time you are looking to travel.**

Ask the recruiter what hours she is available. The answer should be that someone from the company is available to help you 24 hours a day, seven days week. **It is a must that someone is available, at all times, to assist you.**

Fast facts in a nutshell

A representative from the company should be available around the clock.

It is important to find out if the company has a permanent division and/or a local registry division. The permanent division may help you find a position at a hospital in which you might want to permanently relocate. A staffing company that also has a registry division may come in handy if you want to pick up extra shifts at different facilities or want to try out an area for a short period of time.

Write down the answers from each company "interview" and compare the results. Make a list of the benefits and qualities that are important and compare those to the results of the interviews. Find the two or three companies that closely match your "most important" list. These are the companies to which you will want to apply and begin the paperwork process.

Fast facts in a nutshell

Compare recruiter interview results to choose a company to travel with.

NURSE INTERVIEW

Now you know what to ask the recruiter, but what will the recruiter ask you? **The first time you contact the recruiter, she will want some basic information,** so the answers will be easy. **This will include your specialty, years of experience, current practice, and desired location.** Then, she will ask to send you an information packet that will contain an application, background check consent form, reference request, HIPPA review and test, fire safety information, and physical assessment form. Other various forms and tests may accompany these. Information regarding company benefits will be included in this packet.

INFORMATION PACKET

After the first few contacts with recruiters, you'll have what to say and ask down pat. **Don't worry about the forms.** Your binder, which you have already compiled, should contain everything you need to complete them.

The tests, however, must be taken. It is just part of the process. The good news is that **the tests are usually not required to start the assignment search and should have study guides attached.** This leaves time to search for the perfect assignment before diving into each company's required test material. It also never hurts to ask if a company can accept another company's tests. Most will not, as JHACO has rules about several of the tests given.

Fast facts in a nutshell

An information packet will be sent from the travel company that contains multiple forms and guides, along with tests and other information.

The travel company recruiter will request that you fill out a skills checklist for each area of nursing in which you currently practice or have practiced during the last year. These can usually be completed online.

The checklists are comprehensive and area specific. **Be honest about what you are and are not capable of doing.** It's okay if you are not 100% proficient in each and every skill on the checklist. **Always ask for help to complete a task about which you are not sure.** This will allow you to become proficient in the skill while keeping your patient, as well as your license, safe.

Fast facts in a nutshell

Skills checklists should be completed with competencies accurately documented.

ADDITIONAL TIPS TO EASE FINDING AN ASSIGNMENT

Once you pick a company, tell the recruiter your desired specialty or specialties (if you have more than one), desired location, and preferred shift. She might have an assignment that fits the bill, and she may also have some alternatives available. **It's a good idea to explore all the options to ensure that you are not missing out on a fantastic opportunity.** Occasionally, two companies will have the same assignment available. Pick the one that offers benefits that suit you best.

If the assignment you are looking for is not available, you may need a change of location, shift, time of assignment, or company. Other companies might have the assignment you want or the assignment may just not be available. For example, in Hawaii it is usually easier to find available shifts in the summer than in the winter, but in Arizona, it is often easier to plan for an assignment in the winter. Your recruiters and other travelers will be able to help you plan where to go and when.

Fast facts in a nutshell

Check with multiple companies and other travelers to find the right assignment at the right time.

PROBLEMS WITH A RECRUITER

The recruiter will be there to guide you through the processes that will ensure your assignment is an amazing adventure.

Rarely, the recruiter assigned to you is not the right match. Read Case Studies 2.1 and 2.2 to explore examples of how to handle this situation.

CASE STUDIES: HANDLING RECRUITER DIFFICULTIES

CASE STUDY 2.1   Savannah's Approach

Savannah has contacted the XYZ travel staffing company, and Ellen is her recruiter. Savannah is a critical care nurse with 12 years of experience. She would like to take an assignment in California working the day shift. She has three children and wants to take them on assignment with her this summer. XYZ has all the benefits Savannah desires.

Ellen is a seasoned recruiter and really wants to fill the severe needs portion of the company's roster. She informs Savannah that there are critical care assignments in California this summer, but most are on the night shift. Ellen encourages her to interview and accept a night shift position, even though her children will be coming along. Savannah becomes confused about the situation and feels uncomfortable about the pressure she is receiving from the recruiter.

Savannah accepts an assignment in Los Angeles that is a 7 PM to 7 AM shift. She leaves her children at her home locale, with their grandmother, because she feels she cannot properly care for them while alone and working a night shift. She misses her kids and becomes unhappy with her assignment. She didn't enjoy her 13 weeks in California at all.

CASE STUDY 2.2   Katie's Approach

Katie has also chosen to travel with company XYZ. She is an ER nurse who wants to travel with her dog to Colorado. She is flexible on what shift she works. Ellen is also her recruiter.

Ellen still wants to fill her company's severe need areas. She has a day shift position in Boulder available for Katie, but there is no local housing in the area that will accept a 40-pound dog. She encourages Katie to take the position and leave her dog at home.

Katie tries to discuss taking her dog on the assignment in Boulder, but Ellen states there is just not any housing available and doesn't offer any other options. Katie contacts XYZ's operator and asks to speak with a different recruiter.

Tom, another XYZ recruiter, listens attentively as Katie explains her situation. He agrees that there is not housing available for a traveler with a 40-pound dog in Boulder. However, he informs Katie of an ER position, offering 12-hour nights in Denver, where an apartment that accepts pets is available.

Katie interviews, accepts the assignment, and she and Spot hike, run, and play the entire summer in Denver. They both have a fantastic experience.

Lessons Learned from the Case Studies

These case studies demonstrate that **it is okay to ask for a different recruiter if you are uncomfortable with the one assigned to you.** Ask the operator at your chosen travel company for another recruiter or ask to speak with your recruiter's supervisor. Explain to him or her why you are dissatisfied. They will make the proper resolution. The staffing companies want you to take assignments with them and will do their best to help you make the right decisions.

Fast facts in a nutshell: summary

Choosing a travel staffing company is a major decision. When interviewing with the company, use the questions in this chapter to obtain information about pay, as well as about such benefits as insurance and housing. The recruiter will, in turn, ask you questions about your nursing practice.

Chapter 3

Choosing the Right Location and Proper Housing for Your Assignment

INTRODUCTION

You are organized and have chosen two or three companies that fill your needs. The next step on the path to becoming a travel nurse is to find a location for your first assignment. You should consider many factors when making this decision, including the issue of temporary housing when you arrive at your location. Chapter 3 will guide you to the right spot and explain your housing options.

In this chapter, you will learn:

1. How to determine a location for each assignment.
2. The options for temporary housing while on assignment.
3. The pros and cons of each type of temporary housing.
4. The definition of housing subsidy.

CHOOSING A LOCATION

For most nurses, **the two biggest factors in determining an assignment location are pay and adventure.** Some states pay much more than others. As with everything else, the higher the demand, the higher the pay. Several states have active nursing unions that allow for better pay and benefits for staff nurses, as well as travelers. States on the West Coast have laws that govern nursing ratios and pay, so these assignments usually have a higher rate of pay.

Keep in mind that **if the pay is higher, there is a reason for it.** It may be that the position is hard to fill because of patient load, acuity, location, or specialty. It might also mean that the working conditions are difficult.

Fast facts in a nutshell

Pay rates can vary with location, acuity, and specialty.

Finding adventure is easy in most locations. Check to see what kinds of activities are in the area that you will enjoy. Sightseeing, sports, arts, diversity of cuisine, shopping, hiking, and fishing . . . the possibilities are limitless. **Seeking out venues that peek your interest will help uncover locations that will be exciting.** But don't pick assignment locations based just on what you think will be fun. **Try out new and different locations that will offer challenging activities** and broaden you horizons.

Of course, income and adventure are not the only things to consider when choosing a locale. **Other important factors include the setting (city versus country), weather, family proximity, time of year, and ease of getting to a location.** For the first assignment, an area that is exciting, fun, and also somewhat close to home might work best. The proximity allows familiarity of location, with access to familiar faces. Of course, some nurses will crave a far-off adventure. This will result in a location that provides a huge change in environment and lots of entertainment.

You should also **consider how you will travel to the assignment locale.** Can you drive or is a flight required? With all the airline restrictions these days, this is something to think about. Finally, **consider the kind of nursing you would like to practice.** A rural area may have a small hospital but treat challenging and diverse patient care sets. An urban facility might offer extremely specialized nursing care areas. Choose what is best for you.

The choice of location is important, as "the world is your oyster." A final decision doesn't have to be made just yet. **Once you have chosen a company and a helpful recruiter, check the availability of locales versus nursing needs.** This will help hammer out a destination for your first assignment.

TYPES OF TEMPORARY HOUSING

Housing options vary among companies and are an important consideration when choosing an assignment. Exhibit 3.1 lists the major types of temporary housing used by travel nurses.

**EXHIBIT 3.1   Types of Temporary Housing Used
by Travel Nurses**

1. Staffing company-provided housing options
   a. Private one-bedroom apartment
   b. Shared apartment/house
2. Self-arranged housing options
   a. Apartment/house
   b. Rooming with family/friend
   c. Recreational vehicle

STAFFING COMPANY-PROVIDED HOUSING OPTIONS
Private Housing

Most companies will offer a fully furnished one-bedroom apartment with each contract. Some may include a washer and dryer. A rare contract might even include linens and dishes.

Individual housing is the option most travelers choose. It is easy and economical. If you are traveling with family, significant others, or a pet, this choice might be ideal. However, private housing can be lonely if you are going on assignment by yourself.

Fast facts in a nutshell

A private one-bedroom apartment is the most common type of staffing company provided housing. Shared housing is rare and an upgrade might be available.

Shared Housing

Once in a while, an assignment will only offer shared housing. **This is a two-bedroom apartment, or house, shared by two nurses of the same sex.** Each has a private bedroom, but both parties use the common areas. A great perk of this option is that the roommate assigned to the apartment may become your best friend. The biggest drawback to shared housing is that you'll be living with a stranger.

If an assignment you truly desire offers shared housing and that makes you uncomfortable, ask the recruiter if an upgrade to private housing is available. A nominal fee may be incurred, but it might be worth that fee to avoid the problems that can arise with an unknown roommate.

The housing provided by the travel company is generally close to the hospital where you will be working. At times, a longer drive may be required due to availability of suitable living arrangements.

Be sure to get all the specifics about housing from the travel company housing coordinator for each assignment before arriving at the location. This will lessen the chance of surprises.

SELF-ARRANGED HOUSING
Subsidy Payments

Several options for housing are available other than company-provided apartments. If you would like to find your own housing, know someone in the area to room with, or have a recreational vehicle (RV), a subsidy will be available from the staffing company. The amount varies from state to state and city to city. The higher the cost of living in an area, the higher the subsidy should be. Generally, **the monthly subsidy is comparable to the cost of obtaining housing for you by the staffing company.**

The time to **discuss the amount of the subsidy is when you are obtaining the initial details of an assignment.** If the amount seems low, ask the recruiter for an increase. The worst thing he can say is "no." If the amount remains too low for the location, this assignment might not be right for you at this time. Check on other assignments in the area desired, as the subsidy amount may be controlled in part by the facility.

Clarify how and when the subsidy is paid before accepting the assignment. Ask how the subsidy is taxed. This will be important on April 15th. It is a good idea to **discuss the taxes on a housing subsidy with your accountant** before an assignment is chosen, because the level of taxation is different depending on how the subsidy is paid by the company.

Fast facts in a nutshell

A housing subsidy payment is provided by the staffing company when a nurse chooses to provide his or her own housing.

Self-Arranged Apartment or House

Arranging for your own apartment or house is okay if you want the responsibility. Keep in mind that most leasing companies and/or individual owners do not offer short-term leases. It is also hard to preview the apartment if you are not in the area prior to beginning of the assignment. **This housing option requires a lot of hard work on the part of the travel nurse.**

Rooming with Family or Friends

Sharing a residence with a family member or friend living in the assignment locale can be easy, fun, and cost effective. Be sure to **respect their home and rules.** Try not to overstay your welcome.

The Recreational Vehicle Option

Taking a RV on assignment can be a fun and economical way to enjoy travel nursing. The ability to sightsee along the way, while staying in your own "home," brings a sense of stability to traveling. There are a few downsides, however. The living quarters are small and not all hospitals have RV parks in close proximity.

HOUSING FYI

Whichever type of housing you choose, remember that it can be changed for the next assignment. You are not locked in beyond the end date of the current assignment. There are also a few more things to remember regarding housing.

    If call is part of an assignment, be sure to remind the housing coordinator who is arranging your company hous-

ing. Second, if you decide to provide your own housing or use a RV, be sure the location is close enough to get to the facility in the allotted travel time for a call-in. Remember that traffic varies greatly during the day. Allow enough time to be punctual in arriving at the facility. **Check with the staff at your assignment location for advice about traffic.**

Fast facts in an nutshell: summary

When choosing an assignment location, consider such factors as income, opportunities for exploration, and housing. Housing can be company-provided or self-arranged. Each has its own advantages and drawbacks. A housing subsidy is provided to nurses who arrange and manage their own housing while on assignment.

Chapter 4

"Island" Nursing

INTRODUCTION

As discussed in Chapter 3, the travel nurse has many location options. One extremely popular choice is "island" nursing. And why not? A location in a tropical setting with interesting locals, tons of sunshine, and amazing adventures sounds like the perfect place to practice nursing. While it will be a fantastic experience, this type of assignment requires patience and poise from the nurses who are fortunate enough to fill these temporary positions.

This chapter explains the planning required for a travel nursing assignment at an island locale in the United States and abroad. The pros and cons of this type of assignment will also be discussed.

In this chapter, you will learn:

1. The planning required to practice travel nursing on an island in the United States or overseas.
2. The pros and cons of an "island" travel nurse assignment.

PLANNING

Attempting to secure a nursing assignment that will be either on a U.S. island or an island under another country's authority requires more planning than most other assignments. **There are several things to consider at the beginning of the search for this type of temporary position.**

The first is the choice of travel staffing company. **Most companies will offer assignments in Hawaii and Alaska when one is available.** While the state of Alaska is not an island, it is listed here because of its remote location and the difficulties involved in arranging an assignment there.

Very few companies offer assignments in Australia, New Zealand, or the Caribbean and other international islands. If you would like to travel to any of these locations, question the staffing companies about the availability of assignments for each location. Appendix C lists several travel staffing companies, along with their contact information.

The next step in planning an "island" assignment is to consider the amount of time required to obtain a nursing license and/or work permit for the specific location. Obtaining a work permit to practice nursing in most Caribbean islands, other international islands, or Australia and New Zealand takes substantially longer than receiving a nursing license in Alaska, Hawaii, or the U.S. Virgin Islands.

To obtain a work permit or visa to nurse internationally you must submit several documents, including statements of health, and meet multiple other requirements. It may take several weeks, possibly months, to compile all the information. However, the requirements to obtain a nursing license in Alaska, Hawaii, or the U.S. Virgin Islands are similar to those on the mainland. The steps required to apply for and receive a nursing license in the United States and abroad are detailed in Chapter 5.

When considering an island assignment, consider the remoteness of the area. The type of transportation to the location, along with the things you will need to transport with you, may vary according to the access available to the area. **The more remote the location, the lower the chance for modern conveniences.** Almost every travel nurse desires to take an assignment on an island, or in Alaska, at some point in his traveling career. **The whole "island" idea is enticing.** Travel nursing is the perfect opportunity to explore these fantastic locales regardless of the loss of convenience. You might even discover you actually enjoy "roughing" it.

Fast facts in a nutshell

Planning, preparation, organization, and research are all necessary when considering an "island" location for a travel nurse assignment.

The high level of interest in these assignments makes them difficult to obtain. Interviewing for these positions is extremely competitive, but a few things can help make you a more desirable candidate.

First, and most important, **be flexible.** Let the staffing company and facility know if you have experience in several different areas of nursing. If the desired shift is not available, try another one. Look for an assignment during the least popular season. For example, explore Hawaii in the summer or Alaska in the winter. Both places have fabulous activities year round and might offer a contract extension lasting into the next season. Sometimes the exact location desired is not open. If that occurs, ask about another locale that is similar. The more options explored, the more likely you will be to receive an assignment in one of these exotic locations.

Fast facts in a nutshell

Flexibility is key when an "island" is the desired assignment locale.

THE PROS AND CONS OF "ISLAND" NURSING

The island experience has a lot to offer. Accepting a travel nurse assignment at a beautiful, sunny, sandy locale can be a dream come true. The turquoise blue waters beckon as the gentle breeze blows through your hair. The mountains offer fantastic hiking and breathtaking views. The waterfalls are spectacular, and the local cuisine makes your mouth sing. The fishing is amazing. Many local residents are friendly, interesting, and lively. There are quirky little shops and authentic native finds everywhere. Most apartments have a terrific view, and the smell of the sea permeates the entire place. The job is rewarding, and the nurse manager is understanding. A high number of coworkers are helpful, fun, and friendly.

This is the experience all nurses hope to receive from an "island" assignment and, for the most part, it is what they get.

Working as a traveler on an island will be one of the most rewarding and satisfying times of your nursing career. However, a few myths should be dispelled. This will allow for a realistic view of an "island" assignment and help ensure that the experience goes well.

Fast facts in a nutshell

Maintain a realistic outlook when considering an "island" assignment.

The weather is fantastic, but can vary greatly. Be prepared for rain, some cold air, and bugs. Use lots of sun block. Pack good walking shoes, as transportation might be limited. It is an island; sooner or later you will have seen it all. Note your favorite activities, and repeat them. Try out the local spots, as well as the tourist highlights.

Fast facts in a nutshell

Be prepared and plan ahead when accepting an assignment in a remote area.

The local residents will be interesting, but may be a challenge at times. Remember, this is their home, and you are a guest. The food will be amazing and different. Keep an open mind; try it all.

The housing might be less than ideal. The place will probably be small, but cozy. Most may not offer air conditioning, as the islands should have an adequate breeze. The location of your housing maybe farther from the facility than usual because of the limited availability of suitable living quarters. The furniture will likely be dated. **Shipping costs are expensive in these exotic locales,** and most items are used for many years.

The shops will be quaint and interesting. Local goods will be plentiful. High fashion and varied items may be lacking. Again, it costs a lot to transport goods to an island.

Fast facts in a nutshell

Island housing and the fashions might not be five star, but the atmosphere, food, and shopping will more than compensate for the lack of trendiness.

The actual hospital may be up to date, but it might also be technically disadvantaged. Be prepared for challenges with patient compliance. **Several native cultures still have difficulty conforming to modern medical practices.** The nurse manager will be understanding, but she will have high expectations. **Your coworkers will be thankful for your help, but expressing it may be another story. Give them some time** to get to know, value, and trust you, as well as the nursing skills that you possess.

An "island" travel assignment is an adventure of the body, mind, and soul. It is rewarding and challenging; an experience that should not be overlooked.

Fast facts in a nutshell: summary

Proper planning, preparation, and organization, as well as a positive outlook, will ensure that a travel nursing assignment at an "island" facility is a fabulous adventure. A few challenges may arise, but these can easily be overcome with patience and perseverance.

Chapter 5

Obtaining State Nursing Licensure and/or an International Work Permit

INTRODUCTION

A travel nurse practices in many states and possibly several countries, each of which requires a license. Chapter 5 provides the instructions to apply for nursing licensure in the 50 United States, as well as the basic information needed to apply for a work permit to participate in the nursing profession abroad.

Several U.S. states have joined the Nursing Licensure Compact, or NLC, which has made taking assignments in those states somewhat easier. The rules of the NLC are detailed in Exhibit 5.3.

In this chapter, you will learn:

1. How to apply for individual state nursing licensure.
2. The details pertaining to the Nursing Licensure Compact.
3. The information required to apply for a work permit to practice nursing internationally.

INDIVIDUAL STATE NURSING LICENSURE

To practice in one of the United States, a nurse must acquire a state nursing license. This is sometimes easier said than done. All states offer reciprocity when it comes to issuing a nursing license. This means a nurse with a current license in good standing in at least one state can receive a nursing license in another state without taking an examination. In addition to a current license, each state has its own requirements that must be met prior to the issuance of a reciprocal nursing license. Answer the questions in the true/false text in Exhibit 5.1 to gain a deeper understanding of the information required to obtain a state nursing license via reciprocity.

Fast facts in a nutshell

States offer reciprocity regarding nursing licensure.

Most staffing companies will supply a packet of information pertaining to your desired assignment state that will list required documents, how to complete the application process, and the cost of obtaining the license. If additional information is needed, check the State's Board of Nursing Web site (see Appendix D). A step-by-step description of the application can usually be found along with contact information for that particular board.

The cost of each license can range from $40 to more than $150. Additional costs incurred to obtain a nursing license via reciprocity include charges for background checks, fingerprinting, license verifications, nursing education verification, and required continuing education. Check with your recruiter regarding reimbursement. If none is made, keep the receipts to deduct the cost at tax time.

EXHIBIT 5.1   State Nursing Licensure: True/False Exercise

For each question, answer either true or false.

1. Proof is required from the state in which a nurse received his or her original licensure when applying for a nursing license in other states. _____
2. Fingerprinting will not be required prior to receiving a nursing license. _____
3. A background check, with FBI clearance, will be required by every state prior to issuing a nursing license. _____
4. Proof of the completion of an approved nursing curriculum is needed for every state nursing license. _____
5. Your recruiter and the Internet are good places to find information pertaining to required documentation for nursing licenses. _____
6. Continuing education will not be required. _____
7. Most states ask that a 2″ × 2″ photograph accompany a state nursing license application. _____

Answers to True/False questions: 1. True, 2. False, 3. False, 4. False, 5. True, 6. False, 7. True. See Exhibit 5.2 for a clarification of the answers.

Fast facts in a nutshell

Several documents will be required when you apply for state nursing licensure. Determine which ones you will need and gather them in your binder. The cost of applying for state nursing licensure can vary from $40 to $300 (total costs incurred). Contact information for each State Board of Nursing is listed in Appendix D.

HOW TO OBTAIN STATE REQUIRED DOCUMENTS

It will be necessary to obtain the documentation requested by each state before you can receive a license by reciprocity. The requirements for each state's nursing license can vary greatly. Check with your recruiter and the State Board of Nursing as early as possible to learn the specific requirements needed to obtain a nursing license via reciprocity. This will allow adequate time to gather the material before assignment initiation. Once all the information is compiled, send each document to the address specified by the State Board of Nursing. Be sure to request a signed return receipt, so that you will have verification that the material was sent in a timely manner. If an organization must send the document directly, clearly note the address to which the material should be sent. Exhibit 5.2 mentions some of these documents and how to obtain each.

**EXHIBIT 5.2   Examples of State Board of Nursing
Requested Documentation**

---

1. Current nursing license verification. Request this via your State Board of Nursing Web site or by telephone. The fee is approximately $20.00 to $40.00.
2. Verification of original nursing license. Request this credential from the State Board of Nursing that issued your first nursing license. This may be different than your current state of licensure. The cost, again, is approximately $20.00 to 40.00.
3. Background check. Completing this should be as easy as signing a release form from the State Board of Nursing. The cost, if any, is nominal.
4. FBI clearance. This involves filling out the paperwork sent by the State Board and forwarding it to the FBI, along with a fee of approximately $25.
5. Verification of nursing school completion from an approved institution. Contact your nursing school for the proper steps to take to ensure that the request is made in a manner that will guarantee the verification is sent to the correct Board of Nursing. The cost will vary from no fee to $40.00.
6. Fingerprinting. This should be completed on fingerprinting cards sent from the State Board at the local police or sheriff's station. The procedure costs approximately $20. Call the station, in advance, to arrange an appropriate time.
7. Photograph. A 2″ × 2″ photograph, similar to a passport photo, will be needed. No self-taken digital pictures will be accepted. The cost varies from $7.50 to $15.00 depending on where the photo is taken. Local drugstores, some U.S. Post Offices, and various other stores offer this service. Consult your telephone directory under passport services to find a location.

(continued)

8. Continuing education. A few states have certain classes, such as HIV education and child abuse reporting, that must be completed before a reciprocal nursing license will be issued. The Board will notify you if the class is needed and provide a venue for the class to be taken. It is often completed via the Internet or on a DVD. The fee will vary according to the venue, ranging from $20.00 to $85.00.
9. Various other requirements. There maybe some additional requirements not mentioned. Be assured that the State Boards of Nursing will notify you of any additional requirements and provide information regarding how to fulfill them.

Occasionally, a temporary license will be issued until all documentation can be completed. This policy, however, varies greatly among the State Boards and should not be relied upon, as basic requirements must still be met to obtain the temporary license.

> ### Fast Facts in a nutshell
>
> A temporary nursing license, which has its own prerequisites, may be an option until a permanent license is received.

NURSING LICENSURE COMPACT

The Nursing Licensure Compact, or NLC, is an agreement that applies to several states. **It allows a nurse who holds a** license in one of the NLC states to practice in another NLC state without obtaining that second state's nursing license.

This is a fantastic agreement. However, to qualify for the NLC, the nurse must be a resident of the NLC state in which she or he holds a nursing license. If a nurse has a license in an NLC state but is not resident, he must apply for licensure in each state where he plans to practice nursing. Exhibit 5.3 shows the states currently participating in the NLC program.

Check with each State Board of Nursing or with the National Council of State Boards of Nursing frequently, as several states have pending legislature regarding the Nurse Licensure Compact. The Web site for the National Council of State Boards of Nursing is www.ncsbn.org.

EXHIBIT 5.3   Nursing License Compact States, as of July 2008, per the National Council of State Boards of Nursing

- Arizona
- Arkansas
- Colorado
- Delaware
- Idaho
- Iowa
- Kentucky
- Maine
- Maryland
- Mississippi
- Nebraska
- New Hampshire
- New Mexico
- North Carolina
- North Dakota
- Rhode Island
- South Carolina
- South Dakota
- Tennessee
- Texas
- Utah
- Virginia
- Wisconsin

Fast facts in a nutshell

The Nursing Licensure Compact applies to nurses who are residents of a NLC state and hold an active nursing license in that state.

OBTAINING A WORK PERMIT

A work permit is required to work internationally. The length of time it takes to obtain a permit varies from country to country, as does the time the permit will last. The requirements for obtaining a work permit are similar for most countries, but the international travel nurse must verify the information with each one, as well as with her employer to prevent the omission of required documents. Exhibit 5.4 lists the general information needed to qualify for a work permit.

Working Holiday Visa

This visa is the most common work permit issued. Other types of permits are unrealistic, particularly since they usually require a commitment of 18 months to 2 years. The working holiday visa allows young, independent travelers to travel and work internationally for a period of 12 to 23 months. **The working holiday is designed for nurses who will be primarily "vacationing" and nursing secondarily.**

EXHIBIT 5.4   Requirements for an International Work Permit

---

1. Passport.
2. Birth certificate.
3. Marriage certificate or evidence of a name change.
4. Active nursing license in good standing.
5. A detailed curriculum vitae.
6. Evidence showing completion of 450 hours of professional nursing practice in the last three years.
7. Reference checks.
8. Academic transcripts.
9. Current background check (within the last six months).
10. An offer of employment in an occupation that is a needed in the country. Nursing usually meets this requirement.
11. A detailed job description.
12. Evidence that you are qualified by training and/or experience to accept the offer of employment.
13. Health and character requirements based on age, job, and length of stay.

Participating Countries

The following countries participate in the working holiday visa program: Argentina, Belgium, Canada, Chile, the Czech Republic, Denmark, Finland, France, Germany, the Hong Kong Special Administrative Region, Ireland, Italy, Japan, Korea, Malaysia, Malta, Netherlands, Norway, Singapore, Sweden, Taiwan, Thailand, the United Kingdom, and Uruguay.

Eligibility

Exhibit 5.5 lists the eligibility requirements for the working holiday visa.

While on "working holiday," you must also adhere to the following guidelines.

1. You must not take up permanent employment unless you apply for and are granted an ordinary work permit.
2. You must follow the conditions of the working holiday visa.
3. You cannot enroll in more than one training or study course during your stay. The course cannot be longer than three months.
4. You must meet certain health requirements and/or provide medical certificates based on your length of stay.

EXHIBIT 5.5   Requirements to Qualify for the Working Holiday Visa

---

1. Age: 18 to 30.
2. No accompanying children.
3. Hold a return ticket or have sufficient funds to purchase a ticket.
4. Meet health and character requirements.
5. Satisfy that the main reason for traveling to the desired country is for vacation, not work.
6. Not have been approved for a work permit under a working holiday visa previously.

> ## Fast facts in a nutshell
>
> A working holiday visa is available in several countries. Multiple restrictions pertain to this work permit.

ADDITIONAL INFORMATION

It is best to have the new state nursing license before arriving at your assignment. However, if it can be picked up in the area or can be verified online, it may be okay to go without the actual card in hand. Double check with your recruiter and the nurse manager at the assignment to clarify what is acceptable.

> ## Fast facts in a nutshell: summary
>
> State boards of nursing offer licensure via reciprocity if all documentation required is received. The Nursing Licensure Compact also allows licensure reciprocity. It is an agreement among several states that allows a nurse to practice in all of them using a single nursing license. A U.S. nurse can obtain a permit to work internationally, although several documents are required and restrictions do apply.

Chapter 6

Bringing Family and/or Pets on Assignment

INTRODUCTION

Bringing a family member or a pet along on a travel nursing assignment can provide both parties with a fun and rewarding experience. However, special arrangements must be made before embarking on the journey. Chapter 6 examines the planning involved in traveling with a companion.

In this chapter, you will learn:

1. How to prepare for bringing a spouse or significant other on assignment.
2. What plans are needed to complete an assignment with a child or children.
3. Restrictions and regulations when a traveler has a pet.

FAMILY MEMBERS

Nurses who travel with their spouses, significant others, or children will enjoy the rewards that having a companion brings. Sightseeing, enjoying local cuisine, shopping, and exploring in the assignment locale can be more fun when you share it with someone you love. However, bringing others on assignment creates challenges.

A spouse or significant other will want to consider his or her work prospects, or lack there of, at the assignment location. He or she may choose not to work or might be able to arrange for a temporary job. Some couples opt to alternate who works on each assignment.

Generally, assignments only last 13 weeks. **After one is completed, you and your spouse will want to reevaluate the situation to see if changes need to be made.** Whatever the decision, remember it must be mutual. When both parties are flexible, traveling with your spouse can be a fantastic adventure that you both will cherish for years to come.

Fast facts in a nutshell

Compromise is the key to making "traveling" with a spouse or significant other an amazing experience.

Taking a child or children on assignment can also be extremely enjoyable. However, several considerations need to be evaluated. Child care, schooling, and health care are important factors. **Be sure to research your prospective area to**

ensure that adequate facilities and resources are available. Make arrangements, as needed, before arriving at the assignment location.

Many travel nurses like to take assignments during the summer months because their children are out of school. This can make taking the children along a much easier task. However, throughout the year assignments can vary in length from four weeks to six months, allowing a flexible schedule for the traveler and his or her children. Extensions and renewals may also exist that could provide for a longer period of time at one assignment locale. With all these options, traveling with a child can be easily accomplished. With the proper planning, **the nurse and children will enjoy the travel assignments, forming bonds and memories that will last a lifetime.**

Fast facts in a nutshell

When taking children on assignment, plan well to ensure experiences that will create lasting memories.

PETS

Pets are incredible companions to have along on a travel assignment; your furry friend will provide pure "creature" comfort. While traveling with a pet, keep in mind that some states, such as Hawaii, have regulations and restrictions regarding animals. **Inquire with the state to which you plan to travel for the specifics regarding Fido.**

Tell your recruiter and housing coordinator, in advance, that a pet will be accompanying you on assignment. This will help them to find a position with available pet-friendly housing. A deposit may be required, ranging from $250 to $500. It can usually be deducted from your first paycheck received from the travel company.

Confirm with your veterinarian that your pet's shots are up to date and bring copies of her medical records on assignment. It is also a good idea to have your pet microchipped. If he gets lost in a new city, the pet can easily be found because veterinarians and animal shelters can use a wand that deciphers microchip information. An engraved tag, located on his collar, showing an accurate phone number is also helpful.

If you fly to an assignment locale with a pet, a health certificate will be required. Check with the airline carrier for specific requirements and restrictions.

Ask your coworkers, once you begin the new assignment, for the name of a good local vet. It's handy to have his number, just in case. Inquire about great places that you and your furry companion can explore. A great adventure awaits the both of you.

Fast facts in a nutshell

Pets make great companions while you are travel nursing, although a moderate amount of planning is required if you are to bring one along.

Tell the staffing company recruiter early if you plan to bring a pet, a significant other, or a child on a travel assignment. In addition, let her know if you want to pair up with a friend who is a traveler. **The sooner the recruiter knows of any special arrangements you may require, the easier it will be for the two of you to decide which assignment will best fulfill your needs.**

Fast facts in a nutshell: summary

Taking a family member or pet on a travel nurse assignment is fun and rewarding. However, careful planning is required. The staffing company recruiter will guide you to the proper position and a location that allows a spouse, significant other, child, friend, or pet to accompany you on your travels. She will also help you manage the planning and paperwork needed.

Chapter 7

Interviewing with a Potential Assignment Facility and Negotiating a Contract

INTRODUCTION

To become a travel nurse, you must accept a travel assignment. An interview will be completed, with a prospective assignment facility, before the staffing company offers you a temporary position. Chapter 7 explains the interview and details the questions a nurse should ask of the prospective hospital interviewer.

After an interview is completed and an offer for an assignment is made, a contract will be submitted by the staffing company to the traveler. The contract will contain the details pertaining to the assignment, such as facility, location, dates of service, housing, pay, insurance, shift, and hours contracted. It should be highly scrutinized. This chapter describes how to examine the contract and how to negotiate any needed changes.

In this chapter, you will learn:

1. How to perform an interview with a prospective assignment facility.
2. What information to expect in a standard travel staffing company contract.
3. How to negotiate changes to the assignment contract.

THE INTERVIEW

Nine times out of ten, **the nurse manager of the potential assignment unit will conduct the interview via telephone.** However, the nurse manager may opt to use an assistant manager to complete it in her absence. On rare occasion, a human resources representative will conduct an initial interview, and the nurse manager will complete a follow up, if needed. The representative may be from the hospital or from the staffing company. This person should not be a recruiter.

Inform your recruiter how and when you would like to be contacted, and she will pass this information along to the appropriate personnel. Most travel nurses prefer to provide their cellular telephone number, as it allows for greater flexibility. Remember that it is okay to use voice mail. For example, if the nurse manager calls a nurse while she is at the grocery store, the call will roll over to voice mail. The nurse can then call back at a quite time when there are no distractions.

Do not be overly concerned if it takes a day or two to reach the manager. Leave a message with a good contact time. If an assignment seriously interests you and a few days have gone by with no word for an interview, ask the company recruiter for the nurse manager's number. It is usually okay to give her a call. Your recruiter will let you know if the manager has asked not to be contacted in this way.

Fast facts in a nutshell

A nurse manager usually conducts the interview via telephone.

The nurse manager has received your credentials, certifications, and profile from the staffing company and has reviewed the information. You were granted an interview because the facility is interested in you for the position. The interviewer will ask questions to further clarify your information and will provide information about the facility, unit, and available assignment. **This interview is your chance to ask questions about this assignment that pertain to the facility.**

Before the interview, **research the facility and the area it serves on the Internet.** This will provide a base of information on which to build. **Have a pen, paper, and a list of questions available when the interview is conducted.** Exhibit 7.1 details the questions that should be asked by the travel nurse during the interview.

One thing that is not necessary to discuss with the manager or interviewer is pay and benefits. These topics will be handled through your recruiter and stated in the contract upon assignment acceptance.

Write down the answers to your questions during the interview, as well as any additional information provided.

EXHIBIT 7.1   **Questions to Ask a Prospective Nurse Manager Regarding the Unit, Facility, and Assignment**

---

1. What are the hours and shift?
2. Does this unit participate in shift rotation? Carefully consider accepting a night or rotating shift if you are currently on days. Think about the change in your sleep schedule, coupled with the other changes a traveler experiences while on assignment.
3. Is call required? Confirm the hours of call, how much call will be required, and the average number of callbacks per week. Make careful decisions regarding an assignment that has call requirements, particularly if call isn't already a part of your routine.
4. What is the patient-to-staff ratio and how often does a deviation occur? Keep in mind that while some states have laws in place that mandate staffing ratios, most do not.
5. What types of resources and staff support systems are available? An example of a good response is that the hospital policies are available on a computer located at the nurses' station.
6. Can days off be requested? This is the best time to clarify days off that may be needed.
7. What is the float policy?

This allows easy recall of the details pertaining to the assignment. It's also easier to compare two assignments side-by-side with the written information on hand.

Fast facts in a nutshell

Ask the interviewer questions pertaining to the assignment and write down the answers for easier recall.

During the interview, do not indicate whether you plan to accept the assignment or not. On completion of the interview, thank the manager for her time and leave it at that. He or she does not expect a commitment at this time.

Interview with a few managers to get a feel for what is available. You don't have to take the first assignment that is offered. **Shop around to find the best fit.** Choose an assignment in an area you desire with a manager you feel comfortable with.

When you decide that you would like to accept a particular assignment, notify your recruiter. He or she will provide the contract details and help you proceed to the next step of your travel-nursing journey.

Fast facts in a nutshell

Notify the recruiter, not the interviewer, when you agree to accept the assignment.

THE CONTRACT

The final step to complete before embarking on a travel assignment is to sign a contract whose terms are accepted by you, the staffing company, and the facility. When negotiating the contract with the company recruiter, be sure to clarify all the issues listed in Exhibit 7.2.

A few more details need to be addressed before accepting and signing the assignment contract. **If you are receiving a rental car or car subsidy, check that it is documented in the contract.** Most assignments requiring call should incorporate this provision. **Clarify who is responsible for car insurance** on the rental vehicle. It is usually the travel company's responsibility to cover the car. However, not all assignments have the

---

EXHIBIT 7.2   Details to Verify Regarding a Travel Nurse Assignment Contract

1. Pay.
2. Call.
3. Days off. If the manager has agreed to honor them, get this written into the contract.
4. Completion bonus and hours required to receive it.
5. Housing or amount and timing of subsidy payments.
6. Insurance.
7. Travel reimbursement.
8. Start and completion dates.
9. Are your hours guaranteed?

---

same policies. If you are responsible for the insurance, a rider from your insurance company may be all that is required. Clarify this with your agent. The rental car companies do offer optional insurance, but it is costly. **Get all the specifics, regarding the rental car, prior to arriving at the assignment locale.**

Is a "float" policy stated in the contract? As nurses, we understand floating to be the practice of reassigning nurses from their usual assigned unit to a short-staffed area. Some travelers enjoy the change, while others dread it. **If you prefer not to float, get it documented in the contract.** This will help to avoid problems later. However, you may find that floating at certain facilities is unavoidable.

Check that the hiring policy with the hospital is noted in the contract. You might like the area and facility so much that you decide to hire on after the assignment is completed. Most companies require that they manage the employment process. That is acceptable. It is just best to know what the procedure is ahead of time.

It is also best to be prepared. Investigate the cancellation policy for you, the travel company, and the facility. This information probably will not come into play, but it is smart to be aware of all possibilities.

Now is the time to clarify and define the contract. Negotiate on areas, if needed. Some companies may provide an increase in hourly pay, or subsidy, if you provide your own health insurance. Others may pay a lower hourly rate and a greater subsidy if you prefer. This can offer tax benefits, in some instances.

Before signing and returning the contract, ask any questions that you may think of. Remember, the only stupid question is the one not asked. Discuss all options available with the recruiter to design a contract that is tailored just for you. Write the answers down to refer to later.

Fast facts in a nutshell

- Confirm rental car provisions, if applicable, before embarking on an assignment.
- Clarify the float policy before accepting an assignment.
- Be aware of your assigned facility's hiring policy and contract cancellation terms.
- Negotiate a contract for "you."

The company will assemble the contract and any additional paperwork needed. It will be mailed, but can be faxed in certain instances. **Once the contract is received, read it carefully. Confirm that every detail noted above and discussed in the interview is addressed correctly.** It is okay to wait a day or two before actually "accepting" the assignment. Take the time to review all the information about the potential assignment that you have obtained and make a secure decision. Your recruiter will understand. Don't worry. Each time you interview, accept, and complete an assignment, it will get easier.

Fast facts in a nutshell: summary

The nurse manager, or her representative, will complete a telephone interview with a travel nurse candidate before the staffing company offers an assignment. The travel nurse should ask several questions during the telephone interview to ensure that the assignment is a proper fit. After a successful interview, a contract among the nurse, the staffing company, and assignment facility will be utilized. This contract will detail the specifications pertaining to the travel assignment and should be carefully scrutinized.

Part II

Keys to Assignment Preparation

Chapter 8

Types of Transportation to the Assignment Location

INTRODUCTION

Preparation for a travel nursing assignment involves several steps, as well as good organizational skills. The first step is deciding how to get to the assignment location. Chapter 8 explores the transportation options available to the traveler, along with tips to make choosing among them easier.

In this chapter, you will learn:

1. The four major modes of transportation used to get to a travel nursing assignment.
2. The pros and cons of each type of transportation.

TYPES OF TRANSPORTATION

Nurses use the four major types of transportation shown in Exhibit 8.1 to travel to an assignment location.

EXHIBIT 8.1   Modes of Transportation for Traveling to an Assignment Locale

1. Airplane   3. Car or truck
2. Train   4. Recreational vehicle

Airplane Travel

Traveling by airplane is the fastest mode of transportation that can be used to reach an assignment destination. Some staffing companies will arrange the flight, while others will simply provide reimbursement for the costs incurred. If making your own reservations, the Internet is the best resource for comparing flights. A travel agent is another good resource.

Airplanes provide for a quick, safe, and somewhat economical trip. However, they also have drawbacks. Baggage rules are strict. Most airlines limit the weight of a suitcase to 50 pounds, usually with a two-bag limit. Certain flights and types of tickets are even more restrictive, such as charging a fee for a single piece of checked luggage. Note the regulations of each ticket carefully before purchasing it. Weigh your baggage before leaving for the airport. This will allow you to exchange items between suitcases or remove unnecessary things. With the restrictions and fees experienced today, vigilance is needed when it comes to flying.

Several nurses fly first class. Here, the weight and baggage limits change, which allows for more flexibility. The cost is higher, but occasionally a one-way, first-class ticket for the same price as a coach ticket is available. This one-way option is also convenient if you are planning to stay at a location for an un-determined amount of time. Exhibit 8.2 details a few more tips that will make traveling by airplane easier and more affordable. The advice will also help prevent delays and frustration.

EXHIBIT 8.2   Tips to Follow for Flying with Ease

1. Check with your chosen airline about all options that are available prior to making a reservation.
2. Arrive at the airport at least 1 hour ahead of the stated departure time for domestic flights and 1 1/2 hours early for international flights
3. Follow airline security guidelines when packing checked and carry-on baggage. This information is available at each airline's Web site.
4. Pack a book, crossword puzzle, or soduko in your carry-on bag to provide entertainment in the case of a delay.
5. Wear comfortable clothing and easy to remove shoes, as it maybe necessary to remove your shoes during the security check.
6. Be prepared for carry-on luggage, as well as checked bags to be manually searched. If you decide to lock the bags, keep a key easily accessible.
7. Call the airline, or check its Web site to ensure that the flight is not delayed before leaving home.
8. Ask if any upgrades are available when checking in at the terminal.
9. If traveling with a pet, verify the airline's pet policy along with its departure and arrival requirements pertaining to the animal.
10. When flying with small children, clarify the child seat versus ride-in-lap policy of the airline.

If you do fly to the assignment locale, verify with the staffing company how you will get to your housing once in the destination city. Most areas have excellent public transportation, but some will require the use of a rental car.

Fast facts in a nutshell

- Airline travel is often the fastest and most economical way to travel to an assignment.
- Baggage limits vary with the type of airline ticket purchased. Read the restrictions carefully.
- Preparation prior to air travel will increase comfort and relaxation, while decreasing anxiety and irritation.

Train Travel

Traveling by train is relaxing and picturesque. It is interesting and requires little effort from you. The view can be amazing. However, **train travel is more time consuming than flying.** Bringing a friend, spouse, or family member along can make the time move faster, though sometimes the quiet is nice.

The Internet is a good place to research options and reservations. Train travel also has restrictions regarding baggage. Check with each supplier for specifications and limitations. Secure transportation from the train station to your housing prior to arriving at the assignment destination.

> ## Fast facts in a nutshell
>
> Train travel can be a relaxing mode of transportation to an assignment destination, but needs to be researched properly.

Automobile Travel

To reach most assignments, driving a car or truck is the best option. The scenery is nice, and the travel time is reasonable. You will also have the flexibility of your own car for commuting and sightseeing while on assignment. If this assignment is eligible for a rental car, a car allowance should be available in lieu of the rental.

Properly prepare the automobile before beginning the trip to your new locale. Perform all routine maintenance and have any needed repairs completed in your hometown. **A dependable car is a must.**

Consult a reliable map resource for excellent directions and follow them. Most online sites provide similar directions, but compare two or three to find the best route. Print directions to and from any sightseeing trips that are planned. Purchase a book containing maps of all the states through which you will be driving. Learn how to read a map if you don't already know. Remember to put the map book into the car. And always ask for directions and help if you need it. Consider purchasing a GPS. They are easy to use and very helpful.

Ask your recruiter or housing coordinator about parking availability at your housing location, as well as at the facility where you will be working. If you have arranged for housing, check with the landlord regarding where it is acceptable to park.

Fast facts in a nutshell

Consult a map often and clarify the parking rules at the assignment housing and facility.

Get in touch with your car insurance provider before embarking on this journey to ensure that your coverage is up to date and appropriate for all the states through which you will be traveling. Your car insurance company may offer a roadside assistance program at a low rate to existing customers. Such a program is an excellent idea. Since several companies offer this program, use the Internet to compare them and choose the one whose options fit best your needs.

Fast facts in a nutshell

Driving a dependable automobile to an assignment is often the best choice. Verify your car insurance coverage before going on an assignment and consider joining a roadside assistance program.

For overnight stays along the way, there are tons of hotel and motels to choose from. They can be found at almost every highway exit. Generally, no reservations are required. However, if you prefer certain chains, specific locations, particular amenities, or bed and breakfast accommodations, reservations are suggested.

Fast facts in a nutshell

Roadside hotels are acceptable places to stay overnight when traveling to an assignment locale.

Driving to a new city is exciting. **Try to allow extra time for sightseeing** along the way. If traveling alone, consider inviting someone to share the drive. Several nurses enjoy having a friend or relative with them to explore, as well as to take on a bit of driving. After the nurse is settled in, the companion will fly back home. Others enjoy driving alone.

When planning side trips, research the opening and closing times of parks, museums, and/or entertainment venues so you can schedule your trip to take maximum advantage of these sites. Check if reservations for specific venues are required. Nothing is worse than looking forward to an event all day, just to find that it is closed or sold out. Remember the Griswolds?

> **Fast facts in a nutshell**
>
> Plan some fun sightseeing trips when driving to an assignment and verify venue times.

To help with any issue that may arise along the road, **a nationwide cell phone service that includes unlimited roaming for "dead" areas is suggested.** This phone will come in handy for all travel nurses and is discussed further in Chapter 10.

> **Fast facts in nutshell**
>
> A cellular phone is a must when "traveling."

Recreational Vehicle Travel

Driving, or pulling, a recreational vehicle (RV) to an assignment location is a great alternative to traditional travel and housing. The perks of driving, such as travel time and sightseeing are enjoyed, plus you can sleep in your own bed every night. Fast food is not required because the kitchen travels, too. Public restrooms are a thing of the past.

When traveling in a RV, plan the drive carefully. Follow the advice provided for automobile travel. For overnight stays, stop at an RV park or other acceptable, safe area. Schedule time for sightseeing. When bringing a tow car, check with the parks in your assignment locale for the availability of parking an extra vehicle.

Fast facts in a nutshell: summary

The four major modes of transportation for traveling to an assignment location are airplane, train, automobile, and recreational vehicle. Each type of transportation requires preparation and has specific guidelines to follow to ensure safety, ease of use, and fun.

Chapter 9

Packing

The Gear You'll Need When You Get There

INTRODUCTION

The next step required to prepare for a travel nursing assignment involves packing. Chapter 9 lists what items to bring on an assignment. The chapter is divided into two sections: personal effects and household items.

In this chapter, you will learn:

1. Which personal items will be needed while on a travel nurse assignment.
2. What household items to pack for use at the assignment location.

PERSONAL EFFECTS

The type of transportation chosen for traveling to the assign-ment location greatly affects what you are able to pack. **Exhibit 9.1 lists the basic personal items needed for an assignment.**

If the assignment is in a warm location, bring appro-priate clothes. Also, pack some cold weather gear in case a trip to go skiing or the like pops up. The opposite holds true, as well. For example, while on assignment in California, there was an instance where my husband surfed one day and skied the next. If the amount of space for baggage is limited you can always pick up any needed items on location. This also pro-vides a great excuse to go shopping.

A good rule of thumb is "if you haven't worn it in the last 3 months, you shouldn't need it in the next 13 weeks." Even so, **it is suggested a traveler bring one "dress up" outfit, which**

EXHIBIT 9.1   Personal Effects Needed for a Travel Assignment

1. Daily grooming supplies.
2. Casual daily clothing (10 sets).
3. Undergarments (7 sets).
4. Robe or housecoat.
5. Pajamas (4 sets).
6. 3 or 4 pairs of terrain and weather appropriate shoes.
7. Uniforms (3 sets), plus work shoes.
8. Backpack.
9. "Dress up" or proper attire outfit, with proper shoes.

---

fits just perfect, along. You never know when a party invitation will arise that requires "proper attire."

Fast facts in a nutshell

Pack daily use personal items, along with 1 or 2 "just-in-case" items, when preparing for a travel nurse assignment.

Clarify with the recruiter what required color of uniform, if any, is needed. It may be best to clarify the color with the nurse manager, as well. This will allow you to bring the right scrubs, if you already own the proper color, or purchase what is needed prior to arriving on location.

Fast facts in a nutshell

Have the proper uniform on hand before leaving for an assignment.

HOUSEHOLD ITEMS

Most housing provided by a travel company is fully furnished. Clarify with your coordinator exactly what will be provided while on assignment. Will the apartment have dishes, pots and pans, a toaster, linens, a telephone, or a TV?

Ask what size bed is in the assignment apartment. This will allow you to bring the right size sheets. If the housing co-ordinator is unsure, one set of full sheets and one set of queen sheets is ideal. **It is recommended that two sets of sheets be packed**, so that you always have a clean set to use while the other is in the wash. Two to three sets of towels, including a washcloth and hand towel, should suffice.

Pack a set of pots and pans if you plan on cooking. A set of four plates, bowls, cups, and silverware will be enough. Bringing a few cooking utensils and some kitchen towels is also a good idea. However, **some travelers swear by paper plates**, paper towels, and plastic cups and utensils. It works for them, as there are fewer dishes to wash.

Ask the housing adviser if a coffee maker, a toaster, an alarm clock, and/or a microwave will be provided. If the answer is no, pack the things that are needed. Most company housing has the basics, but it is best to check it out ahead of time. If you prefer to bring your own things and have the space, that's okay, too.

Fast facts in a nutshell

Ask the housing coordinator exactly what conveniences will be provided and pack any additional household items desired.

Needed items may also be purchased on arrival at the assignment location. Consignment shops, thrift stores, and www.craigslist.com are excellent resources to use to purchase items at great prices.

An example from our traveling adventure occurred while on assignment in Hawaii. My husband and I opted to locate our own housing. Therefore, we had to furnish it. Because we packed only our clothes because of limited luggage space, we acquired all our housing supplies from thrift shops and yard sales. Some of those items were so cool that we shipped them back to the mainland. One particular lamp resides in my current home. Most, however, were donated to a local church when we left the island.

Fast facts in a nutshell

Second hand stores and yard sales are great places to purchase temporary housing items.

It is important to have a computer, a printer, and reliable Internet service. A laptop with a WIFI is a smart option. A printer that can fax, copy, and scan also comes in handy. If you do not have a computer or do not want to bring yours, a library at the assignment location should be a good resource.

You will learn, with each assignment, what is needed and what is not. The key is to make the new place feel like "home" for 13 weeks. We all have certain "creature comforts." Be sure to bring along that special something. Pack a few photographs. Bring your favorite pillow and blanket.

Fast facts in a nutshell: summary

Packing for a travel nurse assignment is easily done with the proper preparation (see Exhibit 9.1). The staffing company provides several housing items. Furniture, appliances, and most small electronics are a few examples. Any missing necessities can be purchased upon arrival at the assignment locale. It is also ideal to bring a computer and a few personal "home" items.

Chapter 10

Banking, Mail, Documentation, Taxes, and Telephones Simplified

INTRODUCTION

Careful organization can help a travel nurse ease the problems that can occur while on assignment. As a result, several chapters, including this one, deal with the question of organization. This chapter specifically covers several areas that need to be addressed before embarking on the first travel assignment. These areas will require maintenance during the course of a travel-nursing career. They include banking issues and handling mail, which require a minimum amount of research to manage properly, as well as document maintenance for personal and professional use, and taxes, which demand a little more vigilance. The good news is that telephone service is easy to tackle.

In this chapter, you will learn:

1. The keys needed to find the appropriate bank to use while working as a travel nurse.

2. The options available for mail delivery while on assignment.
3. How to maintain personal, professional, and tax documentation during assignments.
4. How to choose a cellular telephone company and plan that will provide an adequate coverage area, along with the right mixture of minutes, text, and Internet use.

BANKING

Choosing a bank doesn't seem to be an important decision to some traveling professionals. **Read Case Studies 10.1 and 10.2 to discover just how important picking the right bank can be.**

CASE STUDY 10.1   Troy's Banking Choice

Troy is about to embark on his first travel nurse assignment in San Francisco. Currently, he lives in an average size town in North Carolina and uses a local bank to manage his checking and savings accounts. The bank has branches throughout the Southeast only.

He talks to a branch manager who assures him that he will experience continued happiness with this bank, even while in California. The bank does not charge a fee to use its debit card at another bank's ATM machine. The debit card carries the Visa logo, and the bank will gladly accept direct deposits. Online banking availability, with a bill pay option, is included in the account options.

Troy decides that these banking options are sufficient and begins his assignment in San Francisco without making any changes. During his assignment, however, Troy finds that he would like to

(continued)

makes some changes to his checking and savings accounts. He wants to open another account to manage his retirement fund. He also wants the ability to switch money among the three accounts as he sees fit. Troy contacts the bank in North Carolina. A bank employee informs him that to make any type of change to the accounts he must come into the local branch. Troy explains that he is working in California and unable to do this. The bank manager is contacted but is unable to make the changes by telephone or on the Internet.

Troy is frustrated and waits until he is home, between assignments, to make the changes. He does not open additional accounts with this bank.

CASE STUDY 10.2   Tim's Banking Choice

Tim is also about to embark on his first travel nurse assignment. His assignment is in Los Angeles. He completes some research on the Internet to compile a list of banks in that area that also have branches in his hometown of Atlanta.

Tim learns which of those banks also offer online banking, a Visa or MasterCard debit card, and free checking. He finds one bank that fits the bill. He opens a checking account at the local branch and asks his staffing company to directly deposit his paycheck there.

While in Los Angeles, Tim finds that working as a travel nurse is a lucrative position. He wants to open a savings account. Tim goes to a bank branch in Los Angeles and opens a savings account without difficulty. He is able to transfer money between accounts via the branch, the telephone, or online without incurring additional fees.

Tim saves a bundle of cash. He buys a new car upon returning home from assignment. The loan officer from an Atlanta branch of the bank approves the financing.

Lesson Learned from the Case Studies

Based on these case studies, we have learned that **choosing the right bank with the right amenities can have a big impact on the travel nurse experience**. Banking options, branch location, and online accessibility are just few of the important factors to explore when deciding on which bank to use (see Exhibit 10.1).

A few additional considerations should also be made. Some banks offer debit cards with a points earning system. These points accumulate with each use and can be traded for cash, goods, or services. This is a great perk.

The abovementioned online bill pay option is great for traveling nurses. Bills are paid by computer as you schedule

---

EXHIBIT 10.1   Important Banking Factors for Travel Nurses to Consider

---

1. Multiple branches, preferably one in the assignment location and one located in your hometown.
2. Direct deposit.
3. Multiple account types with multiple options.
4. Online banking.
5. Online bill pay, with little to no fees.
6. Free checking, (may require direct deposit or minimum balance).
7. Debit card endorsed by either Visa or MasterCard.
8. Fee free ATM use at their branches, as well as, at other banks.
9. Changes to account(s) can be completed at any branch, via telephone, or online.

---

them from your accounts. Some banks' bill pay service even applies to bills that do not otherwise offer an online payment option. You schedule the amount to be paid and the party to which it should be sent, and the bank prints and mails the check. It is guaranteed to arrive on time, providing you have scheduled the payment properly. No checks, post office, or stamps to deal with.

If you have chosen a bank that does not have a branch in an assignment locale, **look for another bank in the area that does not charge a fee for noncustomers** to use their ATM machine for a cash withdrawal. This could save as much as $3.00 to $4.00 per transaction. **If a fee-free ATM cannot be located, purchase something at a store and get cash back using a debit card.** No fee should be charged for this type of transaction.

For those of you who may be **traveling to Canada, be aware that not all places accept debit cards.** Most, however, will accept a "real credit card."

While in an international location, the U.S. bank that furnishes your credit or debit card will usually charge a small exchange fee for each transaction. **Ask the banks and credit card companies for their exchange rates.** Try to use the one that offers the lowest fees. Traveler's checks may be a better choice if the bank rates are too high.

Fast facts in a nutshell

- Choosing the right bank, with the right options, in an important decision. Exhibit 10.1 lists the factors that are important for travel nurses to consider when choosing a bank.

- Online bill pay is a fantastic, easy to use, banking option.
- Be aware of ATM fees and debit card acceptance.
- Research exchange rates and fees that may apply when traveling internationally.

The bank chosen by a traveler should fulfill most of these requirements. If one cannot be located that meets all the criteria, pick the bank that offers what you feel is most important.

MAIL

The next issue to handle before embarking on a travel assignment is mail. Because it makes little sense to officially change your address to your assignment location for just a few months, **there are a few options to consider when discussing mail.**

1. Have mail sent to a home address and have a trusted person pick it up and forward it to you at the assignment locale.
2. Have mail sent to the home of a family member or friend, who will forward it weekly to your current location.
3. Open a P.O. Box in one's hometown. A friend or family member checks the box and then forwards the mail.
4. Employ a mail service that provides an address that is a general delivery box or location. The company collects and forwards the mail as arranged prior to departure. The fee

is reasonable and no favors are involved. Keep the receipts for this service in the accordion file set up for documentation maintenance.

It is okay to use the assignment address for a few things, as needed, but remember to put in a change of address with the Post Office to ensure that the mail will be sent to your "home" or primary address once your contract is complete.

Fast facts in a nutshell

There are four main options for handling mail while on assignment.

HOME

What about this "home?" What and where is it? What exactly does "home" mean? Is a "home" required? **There are as many options and opinions of "home" as there are traveling nurses and medical professionals**.

Some travelers keep their houses while traveling. They will have a family member keep an eye on it while on assignment. Some sell or rent out their houses. Many move back in with their parents or another family member prior to beginning a traveling career. Others will maintain their apartments. A number of traveling nurses sell their houses or condos, store the furniture, and go on assignment in an RV. The choice is really yours.

The key is to **maintain some type of "home."** Having a **home base will ease problems with mail, residency qualifications, and the like.** The most important issue regarding a "home" is taxes.

Fast facts in a nutshell

Maintaining a home base will ease several issues a traveler can encounter.

TAXES

Having a permanent tax home affects the amount of tax owed because the fee schedule for taxation varies from state to state. Where the "home" is located may or may not lower the amount you will be taxed. An accountant and/or tax adviser will be able to decipher the tax codes. He or she can provide advice regarding the best decision for you and your "home."

Look for an accountant or tax adviser who has experience with traveling professionals and their special circumstances. Verify that the tax preparer employed is familiar with the federal tax laws, as well as the state tax laws for each state in which you have taken an assignment. He should also know the tax requirements of the state where your have your primary residence.

Working with an experienced tax adviser will save time, stress, and money. Ask other traveling professionals whom they employ for tax advice and preparation. Research these suggestions and look at several options. This will protect you, your money, and your reputation.

The most important thing to do before and after finding a good accountant is to **save each and every receipt while on assignment**. Keep them organized in an accordion folder. The receipts are key to tax preparation and documentation, so save them all.

Fast facts in a nutshell

- Complete a lot of research prior to choosing an accountant.
- Discuss your taxes and "home" with an accountant who is experienced with traveling professionals.
- Save and organize every receipt while preparing for, and during, an assignment.

DOCUMENTATION

Several documents are necessary to bring on assignment. One extremely important item is the documentation binder already compiled. Exhibit 10.2 lists additional things that will come in handy.

94   FAST FACTS FOR THE TRAVEL NURSE

EXHIBIT 10.2   Paperwork and Other Items to Bring on Assignment in Addition to the Documentation Binder

---

1. Driver's license.
2. Social Security card.
3. Birth certificate.
4. Passport.
5. BLS card, ACLS card, etc.
6. Nursing licenses.
7. Health and car insurance cards.
8. Checkbook.
9. Bills.
10. List of contact information.
11. Pertinent medical record copies.
12. Two-to-three month supply of medications, if possible.

A small fire-safe box is a great way to protect the documents that you bring on assignment. Many nurses also put their marriage certificates, mortgage paperwork, life insurance papers, and various other important documents in the box. It is very rare that an occasion will arise when these more obscure items will be required, but it will ease the stress level if they are readily available. The travel staffing company has sent copies of your credentials to the facility at which you will be working. However, some hospitals request to see the actual cards.

A passport will also come in handy. One will be a required at all international land borders, as well as for international plane, boat, or train travel. A passport is fairly easy to get. Go online, download and print the application, get a passport photo taken, and go to your local post office. A background check will be performed and some additional paperwork might be required. Pay the fee for the passport, and it's done. The passport will be mailed once it is issued.

A list of contacts will allow ease of access to important telephone numbers while on locale. The list should include emergency numbers, such as the staffing company's 24-hour contact, the car insurance agent and her company's 24-hour hotline, health insurance contact, doctors whose care you are under, home pharmacy, and any other pertinent telephone numbers. The contact information of the person to notify at home in case of emergency should also be included.

Keep this list on a piece of paper in your purse or wallet. Place a copy in the fire-safe box. Give a copy of the list to your contact person at your home base, too. On your cell phone or PDA, reference emergency telephone numbers as ICE (in case of emergency). EMTs are trained to look for this information after an accident or during an emergency.

If bringing along a family member, also bring along the documents suggested for them. It is especially important to **bring a child's immunization record.**

Bringing a pet on assignment requires a few extra details. You should **have his veterinary records and any required medications.** If flying, traveling by boat, or by train, check with the service provider for their animal travel requirements. **Most airlines require a health certificate from the vet** that is dated within 30 days of the travel date. Pack Fido's favorite blanket, bed, toy, and food. It will make the transition easier for him if there are a few familiar things around.

Fast facts in a nutshell

- A fire-safe box, passport, and contact list should all be brought to an assignment destination.
- Bring appropriate documents for family members and/ or pets along on assignment.

TELEPHONE SERVICE

Travel nurses generally use cell phone service only. Landlines are sometimes provided in company housing and may be connected at the individual's choice. Choosing a cellular phone service is easy. Contact the major companies providing service to your home area as well as to the assignment area, and compare plans. Clarify roaming, Internet, and texting charges. A plan including nationwide roaming for those "dead" areas discovered when driving cross-country is desirable. Choose the plan and phone that best suits your needs.

Fast facts in a nutshell

Compare nationwide cellular phone plans and choose the one most tailored for you.

JUST A FEW MORE THINGS TO NOTE

It seems like a lot of things to keep up with, as well as take along on assignment. **Make a list and check it off as you pack.** Having the suggested items along on assignment will make the transition of becoming a travel nurse easier. You will be prepared for any emergency or problem that may arise.

Most nurses over pack and over prepare for their first travel assignment. That is okay. It's better to be safe than sorry. **You will gain experience with each contract** completed and learn what is and is not needed.

Have someone, at your home base with access to your belongings and paperwork. Be sure that this person is dependable, reliable, and trustworthy. Give him or her your new address, which can be obtained from the travel company housing coordinator before embarking for an assignment. A need may arise for a personal item, or record, from home and this trusted person can ship it to you.

In addition, **give this person your travel route, expected arrival date, and any other information that may be pertinent to your trip.** She can check to be sure everything is going A-OKAY. It's also nice to hear a voice from home upon arriving at your new city.

Fast facts in a nutshell: summary

A travel assignment requires a lot of preparation. This allows an easy and comfortable transition from "home" to "on location." It is important to find a bank with multiple branches and flexible banking options while working as a travel nurse. There are a few options for receiving mail while on assignment, all of which involve some type of mail forwarding. It is best to bring several documents and credentials on assignment and protect them using a fire-safe box. Save and organize all receipts collected during a travel nurse contract. An acceptable cellular telephone service plan will be easily acquired after comparing national service provider plans.

Part III

You've Arrived at the Assignment Locale, Now What?

Chapter 11

Housing Expectations

INTRODUCTION

Arriving at the assignment locale is an exciting and nervous time. The area is new, with amazing places to explore. The sights, smells, and sounds are interesting and enticing. The housing, in most cases, is new and unknown.

This can be a fantastic, yet challenging, time. Chapter 11 discusses housing expectations for the travel nurse who has selected company-provided housing or has chosen to arrange his or her own living quarters. Tips to ease the transition into the new location are provided throughout the chapter.

In this chapter, you will learn:

1. What to expect on arrival at staffing company-provided housing, and how to handled problems that may arise.
2. What to expect from self-provided housing options, and how to resolve issues that may occur.
3. Tips that involve traveling to a locale and living in an RV while on assignment.

101

COMPANY-PROVIDED HOUSING

You have arrived at the staffing company-provided housing. Hopefully, the apartment is everything you thought it would be and more. Usually, **a representative from the apartment complex, or a realtor, will be there to meet you.** The housing coordinator should have supplied you with the contact information to arrange a meeting time.

The representative should perform a walk-through with you prior to releasing the apartment. This is an opportunity to find out how to use all the appliances in the home, as well as to uncover any unexpected problems. **Note damage to the walls, floors, appliances, and furniture. Acknowledge carpet stains.** This will prevent any preestablished issues from becoming your responsibility on assignment completion.

Ask questions about Internet access and cable TV. If you require something that is not provided in the home, ask the representative. If she cannot provide what is needed, call your recruiter. He should be able to help with any needs or issues.

An example of a request happened while we were on assignment in Los Angeles. I needed an extra bed for a few weeks while my mother visited. I contacted my recruiter, who connected me with a housing specialist. A bed was delivered that week. The rental fee, $20.00 a month, was deducted from my check. After my mom returned home, I called the housing specialist, and the bed was removed the next day. It was convenient for us, and the staffing company was a huge help.

The housing coordinator and recruiter will also be helpful when housing problems occur. While contracted in New York, one company-provided apartment was supposed to be "fully furnished." The place had an old, smelly couch, a horrible double bed, and a rusty lawn and garden table set with two chairs. There were no dressers, no coffee tables, and no television. All in all, it didn't have much.

I spoke with the landlord several times, receiving promises that went unfulfilled. After a month, I called my recruiter for help. After explaining the situation, she asked, "Michele, why did you wait so long to call me?" She explained that I should have called her immediately, when the issue was initially discovered. She apologized for the landlord. Within two days, an entire apartment full of furniture was delivered. The recruiter and housing adviser made sure we had everything needed. Now, that's service.

The previous examples show how far a travel company will go to assure a traveler's happiness and provide proper, safe housing. **Let them know, immediately, when a problem arises** and a resolution will come quickly.

Fast facts in a nutshell

- A walk-through will be completed prior to your acceptance of the company-provided housing unit.
- Notify your recruiter ASAP when a housing issue occurs.
- Travel staffing companies generally work swiftly to resolve housing problems.

A few staffing companies house their travel nurses in shared apartments. If this is the type of housing accepted, **try** to befriend your roommate. If issues develop, try to be adults and work them out among yourselves. Exhibit 11.1 provides tips to avoid tension and trouble between housemates.

EXHIBIT 11.1   Ideas to Prevent Problems Among Roommates

1. Label the food in the refrigerator.
2. Arrange predetermined times for entertaining at home.
3. Keep your room, bathroom, and clothes clean.
4. Share the housekeeping duties in common areas.
5. Share the washing machine and the dryer; keep the laundry room clean.
6. Pick up after yourself and any guests.

This list seems full of common sense, but petty things can easily upset a household. **If the situation becomes unbearable and a resolution cannot be found, call the recruiter** or housing coordinator. He or she will act as a mediator to work out something that will satisfy the both parties.

Horror stories abound regarding shared, as well as individual company-provided housing. The reality is that the bad experiences are few and far between. If the company doesn't try to help out with issues that arise, find another one for the next assignment. However, you will discover most companies will do everything possible to make the experience a pleasurable one.

Fast facts in a nutshell

Mutual respect, along with understanding, will make sharing a home a positive experience.

SELF-PROVIDED HOUSING

Travel nurses who find their own apartments or room with someone they know are at a loss for assistance from the staffing company when a problem develops. **A resolution is usually found through family, friends, and/or the local handyman**. If you have chosen to stay with a friend or family member, it might be wise to **review Exhibit 11.1** for ideas to help prevent some issues. Not all the tips will apply to every situation, but one might apply to yours.

Fast facts in a nutshell

Difficulties occurring with self-provided housing are the travel nurse's responsibility to resolve.

RECREATIONAL VEHICLE ACCOMMODATIONS

The RV alternative is an independent housing choice where, again, the staffing company does not provide assistance other than the housing subsidy payment. Your recruiter and/or housing coordinator may know the location of a RV park close to the assignment facility and you might avoid a major RV park disaster by checking with them before reserving a site.

Try the Internet, RV clubs, and RV guides for the location of reliable parks. Some trailer parks may double as long-term RV parking. **Ask other travelers, as well as the hospital representative who performs your interview for ideas on RV parks.** Several of my nurse managers have given great advice about RV sites.

These references provide valuable input, but **always research the park** before locking into a long-term rental agreement or paying a month in advance. Reserve a few days at a time and verify that monthly reservations can be changed without incurring a fee. **It is a good idea to see the spot personally** to confirm that it is suitable for your needs.

Don't be surprised to find **that most RV parks are located outside of major metropolitan areas.** Occasionally, you will luck into one right around the corner from the hospital, but usually **a brief commute should be expected.** A good number of parks will be located along a common bus route, making travel easy if you don't have another vehicle.

Inquire at the assignment facility about on-site RV parking availability. Several hospitals offer this for use by patients and family members only, but it never hurts to ask about the specifics.

Find an RV park that feels comfortable and safe. Full hook-ups have worked best for us, but everyone has their own comfort level. Explore all the options.

Don't rule out the state parks. Multiple upgrades have been made in recent years to accommodate bigger coaches and provide more amenities, with several offering 50-amp service. However, a lot of the national and state parks post a 14-day maximum length of stay. Ask the park host about the rules and how to extend, or renew, the reservation. Occasionally, exceptions can be made on an individual basis. Mention that you are a traveling nurse. It never hurts to let the campground host know that a reliable, working professional is using the site.

While on assignment in Alaska, we stayed at a state park that was absolutely breathtaking. A glacier view greeted us each morning and the site was huge with full hook ups, and 50-amp service.

Fast facts in a nutshell

- Preparation is important when "traveling" in an RV.
- Utilizing an RV on assignment is considered self-provided housing, but several resources are available to provide insight on finding the right park while on assignment.
- National and/or state parks have fantastic campgrounds that are usually suitable for a traveling nurse utilizing an RV.

Exhibit 11.2 lists some additional advice to take into consideration when using a RV as a travel and housing option. Check out a RV guide for additional ideas. Ask other travelers, who have used a RV while on assignment for their advice.

EXHIBIT 11.2 Advice Regarding Recreational Vehicle Use for a Travel and Housing Option

1. Before leaving in an RV, locate the telephone number and address of a trustworthy RV repair shop in the assignment area.
2. Have a reliable roadside assistance program.
3. Prepare your RV for the trip. For example: change the oil, check the tire pressure, and fill the water tank.
4. Have an emergency kit, including flares, available.

A lot of great experiences can be gleaned from others' travels and some pitfalls might also be avoided.

Whichever type of self-provided housing is used, **if the arrangements don't work out for the entire length of an assignment, call your recruiter or housing coordinator.** She might be able to arrange something on a short-term basis. Remember though, if a change is made, the housing subsidy will not be paid for the time company accommodations were required.

Fast facts in a nutshell: summary

Company-provided apartments are generally comfortable and safe. Any issues that occur will be easily resolved when a recruiter and/or housing coordinator becomes involved.

The travel staffing company is not responsible for problems arising at self-provided accommodations. Rely on friends, family, and a local repairman to assist with any issues that develop. Using a recreational vehicle for travel and housing while on assignment is a fun alternative to traditional housing options. Difficulties are easy to solve with proper preparation.

Chapter 12

Getting Settled in a New Town

INTRODUCTION

The housing is comfortable and you've started to settle in. Now, go out and explore a fantastic new city! Chapter 12 is full of information about how to navigate the assignment area, while reaping the rewards of being in a new town. There may be a few challenges regarding traffic and commuting, but these problems are easily overcome. The joy experienced during the exploration of the locale, including the adventures it has to offer, definitely overshadows any issues that may arise.

In this chapter, you will learn:

1. How to use the various resources available for assistance in navigating the assignment area.
2. How to uncover fun adventures, entertainment venues, and the best restaurants in the contract area.
3. How to combat loneliness while working as a travel nurse.

NAVIGATING THE ASSIGNMENT AREA

There are **several resources available that will help you get around town**. The first resource is also the most basic—a map.

A map of the state and general area, as well as a detailed map of the city or downtown area, are musts. The maps will be available locally or can be downloaded from the Internet. Locate a library, grocery store, pharmacy, and gas station that are close by. Use the Internet, ask a neighbor, utilize a GPS, or consult the phone book for a more detailed route to these places, if needed.

Finding the library is helpful for several reasons. Internet access can usually be found and used for free. You can search for things and their locations, then use an online map resource to plot a route. This system will suffice until the Internet at your housing is available.

The library has maps and reference guides for the new locale. The helpful attendants will provide additional information for navigating the area. Researching a sightseeing adventure or finding a restaurant review can also be performed at the local library.

The yellow pages, the Internet, as well as the advice of neighbors and coworkers are great resources for discovering the best places to shop, eat, tour, and explore. Most people are eager to help those who are new in town. Mention that you're a nurse who is helping out the local hospital for a while and advice regarding directions, dining, exploring, and shopping will be endless. Your new coworkers will be happy to help you find places. They will also be a great resource on ways to enjoy time off.

If you experience trouble getting around town, don't worry. It will not last long. Consult the person at work or in your neighborhood with whom you most identify. He or she will provide some tips to help figure things out. One such example is that looking toward the ocean points west while looking toward the mountains locates east. This applies, however, only to certain parts of the country, such as Los Angeles.

Fast facts in a nutshell

- A local map is a must for navigating a new area.
- The local library is a great resource to utilize while on assignment.
- Neighbors and coworkers are fantastic resources for directions and traffic advice.

Each city has it's own tricks for getting around, and once those are discovered, things are a cinch. You'll know this "new" place like the back of your hand in no time. GPS never hurts, either.

EXPLORING AND ENTERTAINMENT

While on assignment, you'll experience lots of new things and, hopefully, learn a few things, too. **It is important to explore the area.** Try not to miss a thing.

Ask your coworkers where to go. Find out what has just got to be seen. Unearth where to eat and shop. You will be amazed at how happy the staff will be to help. People are very willing to share their city and are glad when someone wants to explore it. Ask a few people for their opinion before going on an outing. This way you can get a good feel for the venue before investing your time.

Visit the "local" hangouts, markets, shops, and eateries, as well as the tourist destinations. You can get a fantastic feel for a city if you live like the locals. The things discovered will be wonderfully interesting.

My husband and I found the best brunch in the world while eating with a local hippie dude one Sunday in Malibu. We've since taken several friends there and always stop in when we're out LA way. It's called the Sagebrush Cantina and is located in Calabasas. Check it out, if you have a chance. That was not an ad for the restaurant or a paid endorsement. We just enjoy the place.

Surf the Internet for information and activities in the assignment locale. The **small festivals and markets are fun** and entertaining. This is a great way to get acquainted with the area while experiencing local cuisine.

Long Island, New York, in the spring and summer, has tons of fabulous festivals in its various towns. Catch a few, if you are able. Try picking a pumpkin from the farm, still on the stalk no less, along with wine tasting in the fall.

Fast facts in a nutshell

- Asking coworkers about sightseeing is an easy way to unearth the best adventures.
- Don't forget to try the "local" hangouts and shops.
- Take advantage of local festivals and market days, if possible.

PETS ON ASSIGNMENT

If bringing along a furry companion, **ask your hometown veterinarian if he can recommend a vet in the assignment area**. If the answer is no, a Web search and credential check of several animal doctors in the new locale is a good idea. There will be a few people at work who are also animal lovers, so ask around. These coworkers are perfect for a reliable referral. Research the vet's credentials, no matter how he was discovered.

Fast facts in a nutshell

Research a local veterinarian to care for your animal while on assignment.

Ask the veterinarian, her staff, and other pet-loving folks in the neighborhood about dog parks and pet-friendly excursions. Taking Rover along will allow exploration of parts of town that might have been overlooked otherwise. Use the Internet to locate pet-friendly hikes and venues. **You and your pet will both be pleasantly surprised how Fido-friendly most places are.**

Having a pet along on assignment will provide companionship. You might have also brought your child, spouse, or friend. Maybe you are traveling alone and having tons of fun. All these things do not mean that homesickness won't plague you from time to time.

COMBATING LONELINESS

Combating loneliness can become a challenge while on assignment. Don't let it take hold. Find a new place to eat, shop, jog, or explore. Call a friend. Look through pictures from home and pictures taken during the assignment. Walk outside, gazing around at the fabulous landscape. Try to imagine all the great experiences that await you. If all else fails, call your mom or your dog; these two things always lessen the longing for home.

If you are a person who doesn't mind going it alone, it will be a breeze to explore new surroundings. For those of you who prefer to have a buddy along on adventures, do not despair. **Ask friends and family to visit.** If you have to work a bit while they're in town, you can still try a new restaurant or go for a quick walk in the park either before or after your shift.

Team up with a fellow traveler in your hospital unit or apartment building for an outing. **You might also be surprised**

at how easily you're getting along with your coworkers. They can become great friends who will show you around town, as well as share information on which places to avoid.

My husband and I have made long-lasting friendships with people we have met while on assignment. Using the Internet and the telephone makes it easy to keep in touch. We visit with those friends when we travel to other places, too. For example, we met a great couple in California. While on assignment in Alaska, we joined them in Yukon, Canada. Everyone caught up, grilled out, and had an amazing time. **The ease of friendships on the road is surprising and satisfying.**

Fast facts in a nutshell

Being involved with friends, family, fellow travelers, and/or coworkers can help ease loneliness.

Keep up with family and friends. E-mail is often the easiest way to stay in touch, but handwritten letters, postcards, and telephone calls are much more gratifying. All these avenues provide opportunities to communicate your experiences to loved ones, as well as to share in their daily lives. Find which route works best for you. A mix of all forms is what most travel nurses use while on the "road."

Fast facts in a nutshell: summary

Navigation in the assignment city is easy using maps, the Internet, the advice of local people, and a GPS. Several resources, including the library, will help locate adventures, entertainment, and eateries in the area. Friends, old and new, family, and activity are the best ways to combat loneliness while working on assignment.

Chapter 13

Orientation

INTRODUCTION

Orientation is the beginning of the working part of a travel nurse assignment. This chapter explains the two major types of orientation: hospital and unit specific. The schedule for both types of orientation will vary with each facility, but the information provided should remain constant. These are not going to be the most exciting days of an assignment. Some of the information is required by JHACO, and the rest is given to show an overall picture of the hospital, the unit, and how both function. This will be the perfect time to ask any questions you may have pertaining to policy, procedure, patient care, the facility, the unit, or the patient community.

In this chapter, you will learn:

1. What information will be discussed during a hospital orientation.
2. The purpose of a unit-specific orientation, and what the orientation will entail.

3. What questions to ask of the unit manager and/or preceptor during orientation.

HOSPTIAL ORIENTATION

Orientation should be the first thing encountered on a new assignment. The schedule will vary with the facility. Hospital orientations range from three days to one week in duration.

During the general facility orientation, **a lot of information will be covered,** including hospital policy, protocols, HIPPA regulations, and similar topics. The first few days of hospital orientation may seem long and tedious. It is not an especially exciting time, but it is necessary and informative. Try to get the most from these lectures and speakers. Ask any questions that may come up—even such mundane issues as parking can be clarified during this time.

These sessions occur in a lecture hall or classroom-type setting. Wear something that is professional, yet comfortable for sitting. If you tend to get cold, bring a sweater or jacket. Most of the auditoriums tend to be chilly.

On the first day of orientation, **bring along your binder and nursing license** for the state in which you are practicing. In addition, bring your driver's license, social security card, ACLS card, BLS card, PALS card, insurance card, and any other card or certification that will be used on this assignment.

The travel company should have provided the facility with copies of the cards mentioned, as well as copies of required paperwork. Occasionally, though, the hospital will want something not provided by the company or a piece of documentation may be missing. Some facilities want to see the actual "cards" pertaining to your license and certifications.

A computer class will most likely be included in the orientation. The federal government has mandated that medical records be made electronic by the year 2015 or it will cut Medicare reimbursement to the physician and/or facility. In turn, all hospitals are trying to utilize computerized charting. This makes learning how to operate each system a must. Instructors will guide you through the class by teaching you to navigate the system with ease.

Don't be nervous. Ask questions. **Be sure you are clear on how to use the system.** Learning the proper charting techniques during orientation will provide confidence and comfort when working on the unit. Do not be afraid to ask for help. The hospital wants you to succeed and will gladly furnish additional support to help you achieve charting proficiency.

Fast facts in a nutshell

- An informative hospital orientation, lasting 3 to 5 days, will be provided at the beginning of each assignment.
- Bring your binder, license(s), and certification cards to orientation.
- Computerized charting will be part of the orientation training.

In some states, **fire safety certification is required.** If it is, most facilities will provide the training during orientation. The fire safety class is actually fun. The differences among fires and which type of fire extinguishers to use is taught. At the end of the class, a fire is actually started for you to put out! **Keep track of the certification card given to you.** It is good for several years, which may allow exemption from the training class in the future.

If fire safety certification is required and the hospital doesn't offer it during orientation, ask the orientation staff if it will be offered at another time. Most likely, a class will be coming up at the hospital. If not, the staff should be able to supply a list of times and places where the training is available.

The first day or two of orientation will usually include biological testing. **A urine drug screen and FIT testing for a TB mask are a given.** If you do not have a current TB skin test on record, one will be completed. Some facilities require a two-step TB skin test that may be initiated during orientation. The first step is performed just like a regular TB skin test. The next step is a second TB test that is completed from one to three weeks after the initial TB test was negative. If you've had a reactive TB skin test, the facility will require a chest X-ray dated within the last year. If you don't have a copy, an X-ray will be completed and read prior to your first day of patient contact. These tests should be completed at no cost to you. If the hospital requests payment, contact your recruiter ASAP. She should cover the cost and deal with the facility about payment.

During the orientation, **you will be asked to sign multiple documents.** The forms that will require reading and a signature are listed in Exhibit 13.1. Additional paperwork may accompany the items mentioned.

A test may be given on medication administration, dose calculations, and IV drip calculations. Appendix E of-

---

EXHIBIT 13.1   Documents Expected to Be Read and Signed During Hospital Orientation

---

1. HIPPA requirements and releases.
2. Hepatitis B series completion and/or declination.
3. Facility privacy practices.
4. Hospital policies.
5. Code of ethics.
6. Blood transfusion policies.
7. Medication administration practices.
8. Release for an additional background check.

---

fers a study guide that includes formulas to use for calculations. Equivalencies are also provided. Most hospitals will also provide a study guide before administering the exam outlining the types of questions that will be asked.

Study and be prepared. You learned this stuff in school, and it will come back easily. The facility wants you to succeed. On the off chance that the exam is not passed initially, help and remediation will be available. A retest is then given.

Don't let this test worry you. It is mentioned here to allow for sufficient preparation. The first time I had to take one of these exams, I was very anxious and actually shocked. It had been years since I performed drip calculations. I reviewed the facility-provided study guide and completed the practice test. I was successful, but barely. With each passing exam, my scores improved. Yours will, too.

Fast facts in a nutshell

- Fire safety certification may be required at certain facilities.
- A drug screening, FIT testing, and TB test will be requested during hospital orientation.
- A math test involving medication administration, dose calculation, and IV drip calculations might be given during orientation.

UNIT ORIENTATION

Hospital or "new employee" orientation will be followed by unit-specific orientation. The length of time will vary from facility to facility and may also change from unit to unit. It may even vary from nurse to nurse, depending on experience and ease of transition. A certain traveler might have a weeklong orientation while you may require only three days. This is the time to get as much information as possible about the inner workings of the unit from your manager or preceptor.

The purpose of the orientation is to familiarize yourself with the unit, hospital, staff, and patients, while the staff, management, and patients familiarize themselves with you. This is when you will begin to get comfortable with the new work surroundings and learn the ins and outs of the floor.

Most people you meet will be friendly and helpful, but chances are you'll encounter a few who are not. Overlook those who seem abrasive. They may come around; they may not. This is not a concern. **Your job is to learn everything you can and take proper care of the patients you serve.**

There are several must-dos to complete during unit orientation. Ask the nurse manager for some one-on-one time. Take a few minutes to get to know him or her. **Ask any questions that might have come up in the facility orientation.** She will assign a preceptor who will facilitate your orientation. **Exhibit 13.2 provides several questions to ask** of the manager and preceptor during orientation. The answers will give you a better understanding of the basic functioning of the floor, as well as your place in it.

Some nursing units keep copies of the policies and procedures in a binder located at a central location. Others have

---

EXHIBIT 13.2   Questions to Ask a Nurse Manager and/or Preceptor During Unit Orientation

1. What is my schedule?
2. How often is the schedule made?
3. What is the procedure to request days off?
4. How are changes made to the schedule?
5. What is the procedure for a sick call?
6. What are the penalties for a sick call?
7. How is floating regulated?
8. How is call handled?
9. What is the chain of command in this unit?
10. Where are the policy manuals, including the MSDS sheets, located?

the policies on a computer-based program. It is best to **know
how to use and access the unit-specific, as well as the hos-
pital-wide, policies and procedures.**

If you are comfortable accessing the policies and procedures from their particular location, a check can be easily
completed if the need arises. It is acceptable to ask a coworker
for help, as needed, but **it is also reasonable to refer to the
actual policy and/or procedure manual.**

Always put the proper care of the patient first. This point
cannot be stressed enough. It will protect you, the facility, the
patients, and your nursing license.

**If taking call is part of an assignment, get all the specifics
ASAP.** The call schedule, how any changes are made to the
schedule, the time frame given to arrive at the facility, pager
use, call pay, and call back rules all need to be discussed and
clarified prior to the first day or night of call. Learn how to set
and reset the pager, as well as how to check the alarms, time,
and other various settings. Ask if a copy of the instruction
manual is available.

I made the mistake of not thoroughly reviewing the pager
functions on one particular assignment. The pager sounded
off loudly, at 3 AM the first night of call, awakening both my
husband and myself. It was not the hospital with a callback,
just a setting left on by the previous traveler. Learn from this
example and be sure you know how your pager works.

Having call responsibilities clarified early will ease any ap-
prehensions you might have. Find out how to gain access to
the hospital or facility "after hours." I was locked out once.
The security guard stopped me, interrogated me, and then es-
corted me to the unit in his little golf cart. Okay, you can stop
laughing now.

Fast facts in a nutshell

- You will receive a unit orientation to become accustomed to the new floor and job duties. Asking questions is an essential element of unit orientation.
- Learn how to access unit, as well as hospital, policy and procedures.
- Clarify call requirements and after-hours hospital access during unit orientation.

Double-check the route to the facility from home. Your coworkers should have good advice regarding traffic. There might be a quicker and/or shorter route available. The time needed to arrive at the hospital may vary with the time of day. Try it out before the first shift, the first night shift, and the first call shift.

Fast facts in a nutshell: summary

On arriving at an assignment facility, you will receive a complete orientation that will cover pertinent hospital and required JHACO information. A unit-specific orientation will be provided to facilitate your assimilation on to the floor. Orientation is the best time to ask questions and clarify schedules, call, policies, procedures, and any other issues.

Chapter 14

Tips for Easy Assimilation

INTRODUCTION

The first few weeks on assignment can be treacherous. Every 13 weeks you are the "new person." This designation is the hardest to deal with on the first few assignments. It seems to become marginally easier with each assignment completed or it could be that we just get used to it.

Chapter 14 explains several tips designed to ease assimilation into the new facility. A questionnaire is presented for your completion. After answering the questions, an explanation of each answer is provided to help enhance the travel nurse experience.

In this chapter, you will learn:

1. How to make being the "traveler" on the unit a great experience.
2. How to assemble a miniature notebook that will allow easy access to information required while working at a hospital on assignment.

KEYS TO BECOMING A CONFINDENT TRAVEL NURSE

During the early weeks of an assignment, you will be navigating a new home, town, facility, unit, and staff. **Scary as it may seem, you will get through it with flying colors.** A friend or two will even be made. Plus, the experience gained as a travel nurse is unbeatable.

The questionnaire below, along with the answers and explanations that follow, will provide fantastic tips that will allow you to complete the necessary navigation with ease.

TRUE/FALSE QUESTIONNAIRE
Complete the Questionnaire

Write true or false next to each of the following statements. Then, review the answers and explanations that follow.

1. I will need to prove my clinical competency daily. _____
2. The staff must like me. _____
3. I will be friends with the staff nurses. _____
4. The doctors will not trust me or believe I am competent. _____
5. I should not expect my nurse manager to have an understanding of my unique position as a "traveler". _____
6. I need to know how to perform every procedure without additional resources or education. _____

Answers to the Questionnaire

1. **I will need to prove my clinical competency daily.**

    The answer to this statement is true. The staff, managers, and physicians are not familiar with your background or nursing techniques. **You must perform to the best of your ability each and every day.** However, this is not to say you cannot ask for help. **Asking for assistance is key to providing the best patient care** and an important part of proper nursing practice.

2. **The staff must like me.**

    This one is false. The staff nurses, including the managers, do not have to like you nor do you have to like them. The nurses on the assignment unit will gain an understanding of your clinical competency with each passing day, and you will learn the same of them. This will **provide mutual respect.** Everyone will be working together to complete physician orders, necessary procedures, and provide patient safety.

3. **I will be friends with the staff nurses.**

    The statement is both true and false. Each area of the country, facility, and hospital unit has its differences and similarities just like the nurses working there. On any given assignment, **you will make friends,** and it will usually be with the staff at the hospital. These nurses will share a common interest in the care of patients and that is a good start for friendship. Being open and receptive will also help foster relationship growth.

However, not all staff members will warm to you. There will probably not be a specific reason, and it is of no concern. **Completing your daily work responsibilities in a safe, prompt, efficient manner will earn the respect of most** and is all that is expected.

4. **The doctors will not trust me or believe I am competent.**

   This is false. **The physicians at the hospital will trust the nurse managers to employ and train nurses who are competent.** They also know the staff will be available to assist with any needs that may arise. Be confident in your skills and ask for help when it is needed.

5. **I should not expect my nurse manager to have an understanding of my unique position as a "traveler."**

   This is also false. **A nurse manager should be knowledgeable and understanding** of the unique situation of a travel nurse if she plans to employ one. As a traveler, a lot of issues may arise and support from a supervisor helps to ease the tension. If you encounter a manger who does not appear aware of certain circumstances that are causing problems, approach her in a nonaccusatory manner. She may not realize the situation is occurring. Allow her time to resolve problems. If a reasonable resolution cannot be made, refer to your recruiter for assistance.

6. **I need to know how to perform every procedure without additional resources or education.**

This statement is absolutely false. At anytime during any assignment, **you are permitted and expected to ask questions.** Always ask for assistance from a team member regarding any medication, procedure, or patient care issue of which you are unsure. It is okay to ask for verification of anything that might require reassurance or clarification.

Education should be ongoing throughout your nursing career.

Fast facts in a nutshell

- Use the skills your education and experience have taught, then be open to learning as much as possible.
- Practice to the best of your ability and respect will be earned.
- Enjoy the ease of friendships formed at work.
- The doctors encountered on assignment will trust you and expect confidence.
- Facility and unit management should be aware of, and accommodating toward, the unique position of a traveling nurse.
- Education and support are available throughout a travel assignment.

CHEAT SHEETS

There is one thing that will be a lifesaver on each assignment. It is known as a cheat sheet. This item is actually a small, pocketsize notebook that you keep with you at all times. The notebook will become a mini encyclopedia of each assignment and provide confidence and competence.

The reason it is referred to as a "cheat sheet" is because it will be chock full of notes, lists, tips, and telephone numbers. Convenient access to this information will ease your tension level because it removes the necessity of having to ask certain questions repeatedly. Exhibit 14.1 lists the information you should consider writing in your notebook.

EXHIBIT 14.1   Information to List in a "Cheat Sheet" Notebook on Each Assignment.

1. Telephone list: hospital #, nurse manager's extension and off site contact #, frequently dialed extensions, additional numbers needed in town, and your company's contact information including an emergency contact number that is accessible at all times.
2. Your address, while on assignment, and telephone #.
3. Maps of town and/or facility.
4. Procedural set-up information.
5. Questions.
6. Answers to the questions.
7. Other pertinent information needed.

These little notebooks will be very useful. The "cheat sheet" part comes in handy because a list can be compiled about where to find things, how to get to places in the hospital, or how to set up procedure trays and/or medications for specific doctors' use.

For example, while on assignment in New York, I worked in an electrophysiology lab. Each procedure, and occasionally each physician, had a specific way the tray, equipment, sheaths, and tools were to be prepared and laid out. To avoid asking the regular staff each time I had to set up a tray, I kept a cheat sheet for each procedure and doctor in my pocket notebook. I looked up every procedure until the tray set-ups became routine. This helped me gain confidence because I did not have to constantly ask, "What does he like on the tray?" or " What size sterile glove does she wear?"

Fast facts in a nutshell

A pocketsize notebook containing vital information should be kept readily available.

Clarify that the information in your notebook is accurate. Make any corrections immediately to avoid repeating mistakes. Always **double-check medications with a staff member.**

Keep a list of questions that may arise when the appropriate person to ask is not available. This will allow you to get the "right" answer from the "right" person. Keep the answers in your notebook, along with the questions. The more information readily available, the better.

Please do not misunderstand one point. These cheat sheets will be fantastic, but they do not replace asking questions. **Asking questions is ABSOLUTELY acceptable.** It is the best way to avoid errors.

Perform your duties well, to the best of your ability. This will ensure success and a rewarding travel nurse experience.

Fast facts in a nutshell: summary

To enjoy a travel assignment, perform your job safely and proficiently. Respect the doctors and nurses at the assignment facility. Ask questions when appropriate. This conduct will allow for mutual respect. Compile a small notebook with telephone numbers, lists, tips, and questions with answers to assist with daily work in the unit and decrease the likelihood of repetitive questions.

Part IV

Assignment Problems, Solved!

Chapter 15

Unit Specific Issues

INTRODUCTION

Working as a travel nurse is an absolutely amazing experience. The clinical portion of the assignments will be interesting and offer multiple opportunities for growth and continuing education. The personal aspect allows a nurse to grow exponentially through emotional and physical experiences at work and at home.

However, several challenges may also be encountered during a travel assignment. Chapter 15 addresses issues that are related to the facility and hospital unit. These problems can be overcome when handled properly.

In this chapter, you will learn:

1. How to address personal and patient safety concerns.
2. How to resolve personnel conflicts.
3. How to tackle scheduling problems.
4. How to handle "floating."
5. What to do if you are approached to become a preceptor.

SAFETY CONCERNS

Safety must be taken seriously. **Personal safety issues require immediate attention**. Do the best to resolve the problem yourself. If concerns remain, discuss them with the charge nurse and/or nurse manager. Chances are he will be glad you brought them to his attention and will take the necessary steps to resolve the problems. If the safety issues are not resolved to your satisfaction, notify a recruiter immediately.

Patient safety problems also require a prompt response. Simply asking another nurse to assist in a patient position change will protect you and the patient. If the matter is severe, again contact a charge nurse or manager.

Never risk your own safety or the patients' safety. You are responsible for your license, yourself, and your patients. If an immediate resolution is required and the nurse manager is unavailable or unable to help, contact a house supervisor.

Serious safety issues are a rare occurrence but can happen. Your supervisors and/or company can usually resolve a problem quickly and efficiently.

Fast facts in a nutshell

Address safety issues immediately, and consult the chain of command if necessary.

PERSONNEL CONFLICTS

Personnel conflicts are often easily resolved. Whether an assignment is problematic because of several employees at the hospital or if only one particular person is causing an issue, talk with the nurse manager or immediate supervisor. Calmly and without bias, **express your concerns and feelings.** The unit needs your help. Otherwise, the facility would not be using travelers. Most managers will resolve the situation promptly.

Schedules can be rearranged and unit assignments designed to help ease the distress. Maybe the possibility of being transferred to another floor is available. **Speak up early to prevent discomfort. Call your recruiter,** and let her know about the situation. She will be an ear to listen and a go between, if needed. She might also have additional ideas for a way to deal with the issue.

Fast facts in a nutshell

Notify your supervisor and recruiter when a personnel conflict occurs to facilitate a prompt resolution.

SCHEDULING PROBLEMS

Is your schedule unacceptable or different from what was discussed during your interview and/or orientation? **Discuss these concerns with the nurse manager.** Explain how you understood the schedule was to be arranged. A compromise is generally reached. If the problem remains unresolved, contact a recruiter.

This problem can be avoided by clarifying your schedule, call, days off, and any other scheduling needs, during the interview. Clarify it again when the contract is negotiated. Review the schedule and its policies one more time with the nurse manager or a preceptor during orientation. **Always have specific hours, along with days needed off, documented in your contract.**

Fast facts in a nutshell

Clarification and documentation of scheduling will avert problems.

"FLOATING" ISSUES

Are you frequently being floated to other units or areas of the hospital? The possibility of **floating is something to discuss during the interview and again at the contract negotiation.** Requests can be made not to float or only to float to certain areas of the facility, such as the intensive care units. However, some facilities have a policy that travelers float first. This is often the case, even if the permanent staff has their own float rotation.

If you feel that you are being floated unfairly, talk to the charge nurse and/or nurse manager. **Express the concern**

calmly and effectively. Talk with him immediately, if the clinical area assigned is one in which you feel uncomfortable and unfamiliar. Safety comes first. Contact a recruiter for additional help.

Unfortunately, certain assignments require a lot of floating. Some travelers like the change; others do not. If it makes you uncomfortable, have a heart-to-heart talk with your manager. Most likely, he will find a middle ground that will accommodate you and the house staff. If the problem remains unresolved, punt it back to a recruiter for advice.

Fast facts in a nutshell

Floating is usually a fact of travel nursing, but provisions can be made to make it comfortable.

PRECEPTORSHIP

You are a fantastic nurse who performs the job well. Because of these great attributes, a time may come during an assignment when you are asked to become a preceptor to a new traveler, a new graduate, a student, or a new employee at the facility.

It is absolutely your right to decide whether to take on this role. Preceptorship calls for increased responsibility and a huge time investment. If you enjoy teaching and feel comfortable taking on the extra care and study, do so. If not, explain your feelings to the nurse manager. **Participating in pre-**

ceptorship is rewarding, but it is not required. The manager will understand and there should be no repercussions.

> ### Fast facts in a nutshell
>
> Preceptorship is an honor and can be enriching, however a travel nurse is not required to accept the responsibility.

PROBLEMS THAT REMAIN UNRESOLVED

If you have tried to resolve these or any other issues that plague an assignment and the manger, supervisor, and/or facility managers will not budge—even after the staffing company becomes involved—then you do indeed have a problem. Try your best to arrange an acceptable solution that can at least be tolerated until the assignment is complete.

Thirteen weeks may seem like an eternity when an issue arises, but it is truly a short period of time. It will be over before you realize it. Most situations can be resolved or compromised to get you through. It might just take some heavy footwork, resilience, and vigilance on the part of all parties involved.

Fast facts in a nutshell: summary

Personal and patient safety is a high priority. Any problems with either should be addressed immediately using the chain of command. Personnel conflicts and scheduling issues are usually easily resolved with the help of a nurse manager. A staffing company recruiter is a great ally when problems that occur during a travel nurse assignment are more difficult to resolve.

Floating to another unit is required during certain assignments and preceptorship may be requested, but it is not mandatory while working as a travel nurse.

Chapter 16

Housing Difficulties

INTRODUCTION

An important aspect of any travel nurse assignment is housing. It is imperative that the temporary housing be safe. Comfort and easy accessibility, with multiple amenities and pleasant neighbors, are traits everyone desires in a home. However, sometimes things can go awry. Chapter 16 tackles the problems that can arise in temporary housing locations and how to resolve them.

In this chapter, you will learn:

1. How to navigate temporary housing problems.
2. How to change the housing option utilized for an assignment.

HOUSING SAFETY

Is your temporary housing safe? **If it is not, do not stay there.** Find somewhere else to go, such as a fellow traveler's apartment or a hotel room. **A safety issue must be handled diligently** and is a top priority at work and at home.

The reasons why a location is unsafe vary greatly. It could be that the actual location of the housing is dangerous or that there is toxic mold. If you feel something is unsafe, it is. How to handle the situation will vary with the type of temporary housing chosen.

INADEQUATE FACILITIES

Do you require certain arrangements and equipment to perform activities of daily living? Do you desire additional amenities? **If special equipment is required to complete ADLs, then those particular items should be available.** However, if you would like a bigger apartment, a washer/dryer combo, or an on-site swimming pool, you'll probably have to wait awhile. Again, resolving the situation depends on the type of housing utilized.

DISRUPTIVE NEIGHBORS

No one likes a nosey neighbor, but disruptive and **abusive neighbors are simply unacceptable.** The first recommendation is to discuss the situation with the problematic neighbor. If you feel unsafe in doing so, contact the manager of the apartment, the landlord, a company recruiter, or the RV park staff for assistance. **If there is an immediate danger, always contact the local police department.** When issues with neighbors cannot be resolved, a change of housing may be required.

This will be arranged differently with each type of temporary housing choice.

RESOLVING HOUSING PROBLEMS

Most travel nurses choose to live in staffing company-provided housing while on assignment. This choice makes contacting a recruiter or housing coordinator the first step in resolving problems. **Notify him or her as soon as an issue develops.**

A safety matter should be handled immediately in a satisfactory manner. An ADL issue should be dealt with promptly, as should a neighbor or roommate problem. If an extra amenity is desired, however, a traveler may need to persevere until the assignment is complete and another initiated.

Sometimes, a resolution might involve moving to another apartment. For other situations, it may be as easy as having the proper repair made. Be vigilant about any issues that cause concern. **A resolution should be found** that will put your fears at bay and allow for some sleep.

Several traveling nurses find their own apartments or room with friends and family. **For those who use this option, solving problems is handled a little differently.** If you have found your own housing, speak with a landlord or real estate representative when an issue occurs. Hopefully, they will be able to handle the problem quickly. If not, a local agency, such as the Better Business Bureau or Department of Health, may be a good resource. Worsening situations could result in a move.

If staying with a family member, allow them to handle the issue, unless they are the issue. If that is the case, another type of housing might need to be considered.

If you have decided to hit the road in a recreational vehicle, your options are less traditional. Contact a staff member or the manager of the RV Park about problems that arise. If it remains constant, simply find another park.

Fast facts in a nutshell

- Unsafe housing is an issue that must be swiftly addressed.
- Some housing amenities may be easily changed while others (or the lack thereof) may require a move or another assignment.
- The travel staffing company will help resolve any safety concerns arising in company-provided housing.
- Nurses providing their own housing must also provide their own solutions to any problems pertaining to those arrangements. Allow some flexibility and time for a resolution and you will discover that most problems regarding housing are resolved quickly without too much hassle.

CHANGING THE TYPE OF TEMPORARY HOUSING

Because there are several types of temporary housing to choose from while on an assignment, a change may sometimes be needed. This usually occurs when a nurse has arranged her own housing and, mid-assignment, needs to switch to company-provided housing. A recruiter and/or housing coordinator can generally arrange the change. It will require the forfeiture of a housing subsidy for the remaining contract period. **Notify your recruiter** if you require this change.

Some nurses will choose an apartment from the company and then discover they would like to try another type of housing. When this is the case, the traveler may be required to forgo a housing subsidy for the remainder of the contract due to the arrangements already procured by the staffing company. **Each assignment is different and has its own requirements.** Check with your recruiter ASAP, when considering a housing change.

Fast facts in a nutshell: summary

Housing difficulties arising during a travel assignment are resolvable with the assistance of a recruiter, landlord, RV park staff member, friend, and/or family. The type of temporary housing can, sometimes, be changed during an assignment. Involve the staffing company recruiter when considering a change in living arrangements.

Chapter 17

Personal Emergencies and Contract Termination

INTRODUCTION

This chapter covers two sticky situations: personal emergencies and contract termination. These are considered "sticky" because the definition of a personal emergency varies greatly and contract termination is a taboo subject. However, since this book is titled Fast Facts for the Travel Nurse, *both subjects are discussed and information regarding how to handle these delicate situations is provided.*

In this chapter, you will learn:

1. How to deal with a personal emergency while on a travel assignment.
2. How to terminate a travel nurse contract.
3. If a staffing company or facility can terminate your contract.

PERSONAL EMERGENCIES

Personal emergencies happen to everybody; one might even occur while on a travel nursing assignment. It is best to handle these situations with poise and calmness. **Notify your manager and recruiter immediately and proceed safely to where you are needed.** Do not leave a facility shift without coverage by another qualified nurse to care for your patients. This could risk your license, not to mention patient safety.

The definition of a personal emergency varies greatly, as do the ways to manage it. It may be that you will require a day off to rectify the situation. A week or two might be needed to fully resolve a problem, or an emergency might require that a contract be terminated.

A day or two of leave should easily be arranged with the nurse manager. A week or longer off may require the extension of a contract to fulfill the 13-week obligation. The recruiter easily arranges this, although some documentation will generally be requested. If contract termination is required to handle a personal emergency follow the guidelines provided in this chapter.

Fast facts in a nutshell

When a personal emergency occurs, promptly notify the facility and staffing company to make appropriate arrangements.

CONTRACT TERMINATION

Termination of a travel-nursing contract is a taboo subject. Recruiters and nurse managers do not want it to happen and travelers should **view it as a last resort**. The reason contract termination is not readily discussed is because the facilities depend on a travel nurse to complete an assignment and do not usually have staffing coverage for an unexpected termination.

To discourage contract termination, travel-staffing companies tend to stipulate that **a nurse who ends an assignment early incur some monetary responsibilities**. These details should have been noted in the contract. The amount deducted or due increases for travelers who choose company-provided housing, a rental car, company-paid travel arrangements, or an advance of some form of payment.

The **penalties for early termination should be clearly stated in each assignment contract**. Read all the fine print and take note. It is not common that the need to end a contract early arises but it is advisable to know the consequences ahead of time, just in case.

If a resolution or compromise to an issue cannot be found, and you feel that the only way to proceed is contract termination, try to give at **least two weeks' notice**. Provide this written notice to the nurse manager, the hospital human resources department, and your recruiter. If it appears unsafe to wait two weeks, give as much notice as possible. **Clearly state the reasons leading to the termination**, as well as the attempts made to resolve the problem. **Be sure every attempt has been made to find a resolution** of the issue before termination.

If the reason for ending a contract is personal or an emergency has arisen, the situation is a little different. **Clearly state**

the reasons why termination is needed. You might be asked to provide documentation regarding the cause of the contract termination. If you have it, give it. If not, inform the recruiter and manager that it will be provided as soon as possible.

Fast facts in a nutshell

- Contract termination is a last resort. The terms pertaining to termination are documented in the travel nurse contract.
- Try to provide a two weeks' notice prior to terminating an assignment, in writing.

Most travel companies will complete an interview with you, post resignation, to determine your eligibility to travel with their company, and its subsidiaries again. Someone other than the recruiter will usually conduct it. Present your case clearly. Have documentation available to refer to, if available.

If the reason for the contract termination was a safety issue, you should find support for making the proper decision to put your safety and the safety of the patients first. If the reason was personal or caused by an emergency, again be clear. State your position. Most companies understand that some situations cannot be avoided.

Fast facts in a nutshell

When completing a postcontract termination interview, be clear, state the facts, and provide available documentation.

It is extremely rare for a staffing company or facility to cancel a contract. If it does occur, it is generally before the contract initiation. In most cases, another comparable assignment will be readily available. The biggest reason for facility cancellation is a change in staffing needs. If a contract were to be terminated during the assignment by the facility and/or staffing company, it would generally be due to severe infractions by the travel nurse, such as drug or alcohol abuse on the job.

Fast facts in a nutshell: summary

Personal emergencies occurring while on a travel assignment are easily handled with the cooperation of the nurse, the staffing recruiter, and the nurse manager.

Contract termination should be viewed as a last resort in relation to problem solving. If termination is utilized, provide 2 weeks' written notice. An exit interview will be performed to determine a nurse's eligibility to travel with a specific company after a contract termination by the traveler. Travel nursing contracts are rarely canceled or terminated by the staffing company and/or facility.

Part V

Managing a Successful Travel Nursing Career

Chapter 18

Contract Renewal Versus
Assignment Extension

INTRODUCTION

The first assignment is going famously. You're having a great time! Six weeks have just flown by; only seven weeks left at this facility. What will you do next? Between weeks seven and eight is a good time to start planning for your next assignment.

You might have discovered that you'll need more than 13 weeks to take in all the sights the assignment city has to offer. Or, it might be that the area has really grown on you and another three months in the town would be fantastic. Whatever the reason for the desire to remain at a location, there are two ways to accomplish the task—contract renewal and assignment extension. Chapter 18 explains the difference between the two options and how to negotiate each one.

In this chapter, you will learn:

1. How to negotiate and renew a travel-nursing contract.
2. How to negotiate and extend a travel-nursing assignment.

By weeks six to eight of an assignment, you should have a good feel for the current facility and the area in which it is located. This is a great time to **consider an extension or renewal** of the current travel nurse contract. Your recruiter and/or nurse manager may have already approached you about the opportunity. If not, they will soon, if the facility still has a need. Let's look at a few case studies to highlight the difference between an extension and a renewal of a contract.

THE DIFFERENCE BETWEEN AN EXTENSION AND A RENEWAL OF A TRAVEL-NURSING CONTRACT
Case Studies

CASE STUDY 18.1   Vera's Approach

Vera is a registered nurse from Boca Raton, Florida. Her specialty is ICU. She is currently on assignment in San Diego at a 550-bed facility with six ICU units. The shift Vera works is 7p-7a, including an every other weekend work requirement. She is just completing week 6 of a contract when the nurse manger has asks her to stay another 13 weeks.

Vera enjoys the work but the night shift schedule is exhausting. She has a small dog that loves to get up early to go for walks on the beach. The area is a lot of fun, and there are lots of places that still need exploration. Vera contacts her recruiter for the available options regarding this facility.

(continued)

An extension is offered for 8 weeks, as is a renewal for 13 weeks. She asks for a change to day shift and an every third weekend work requirement. The nurse manger will allow a shift change only if Vera stays for 13 weeks and works every other weekend.

Vera agrees to the renewal for 13 weeks, which allows her to work days. Another contract is created that includes the day shift change. The rest of it remains the same, including the every other weekend work schedule. This new contract will begin six days after the initial one is completed, giving her some time off to visit Los Angles with a friend while retaining her current apartment.

CASE STUDY 18.2   Amy's Approach

Amy has been a telemetry nurse for three years and is half way through her first travel assignment. She is working night shift in rural Arizona at a small 80-bed hospital where she enjoys the staff, acuity level, and patients. The nurse manager asked her yesterday if she would be willing to extend her contract for a few weeks.

After speaking with the staffing company recruiter, she agrees to a four-week extension of the current contract. No changes are needed because the shift suits Amy well, and she has planned to return home for a couple of months after the extension is completed.

Her recruiter faxes an amendment for Amy to sign and send back. The document states the new completion date. Everything else, Amy's shift, housing, hours, and so on, remains the same.

Lesson Learned from the Case Studies

Based on the case studies, we learn that **there is a minimum amount of difference between a contract renewal and an as-**

signment extension. The major difference is the length of time involved in each.

You may choose to extend a contract for 2, 4, or 8 weeks, or longer, while a renewal usually means a complete 13 weeks. **The length of an extension is negotiable most of the time, but renewal duration is generally set.** There are a few factors to consider before accepting an extension or renewal.

Fast facts in a nutshell

A contract extension can vary in length while a renewal is usually a 13-week block of time.

RENEWAL/EXTENSION CONSIDERATIONS

First, are you happy with the travel staffing company? Have they fulfilled their promises and your expectations? If not, it may be time to shop around again for another company. First, let your recruiter know about the dissatisfaction. He or she may be willing to make some changes. Remember, the company makes money when its travel nurses work. They will try their best to keep you on board and happy. If the recruiter or company are not willing or are unable to satisfy your needs, change companies. **Find one that will accommodate your needs appropriately.** However, keep this in mind when changing staffing companies, a full 13-week contract will most often be required from the new company chosen.

Notify your nurse manager of your intention and progress, particularly if you would like to stay at that facility and/or unit. Ask the nurse manager what other companies the facility uses. If she does not know or feels uncomfortable providing that information, check with the facility's human resources, or personnel department, which should have a list of the companies with which the hospital contracts.

You're pleased with the current travel company and love the benefits. Great! But what if you aren't happy with the recruiter? It is acceptable to ask for a different recruiter, if yours doesn't make the grade. Try to resolve any issue with him or her first. If a problem remains, or maybe you two just don't "click," explain it to the recruiter and request that someone else handle your contracts. If the recruiter refuses, or you feel uncomfortable discussing the request with him, speak to another recruiter within the company. It is also okay to get in touch with a recruiting supervisor. Call the 1-800 number, and then ask for the supervisor or another recruiter. Problems with a recruiter almost never happen, but you would hate to leave a company because of one person and that company would hate to lose a great nurse.

Okay, the company and recruiter are fantastic and you are considering an extension, or renewal, of contract. What about the housing, pay, and shift? This is the perfect time for negotiations. If you chose company housing and would like a change or an upgrade; ask for it before signing the new contract or extension. If you live in self-provided housing and would like to change to company housing, or vice versa, arrange it now. The same holds true for a pay increase or bonus.

By extending and/or renewing, you have eased the workload of the recruiter, the company, and the facility. The recruiter does not have to obtain a new person to fill a vacant spot. She does not need to schedule or perform interviews. The company has less paperwork. The facility does not have to provide a new orientation, perform interviews, or train a new nurse. **You have saved all parties' involved time and money** and should be able to negotiate some type of reward for the continued service. The facility must like your performance to ask for continued service, providing a warrant for a reward. A pay increase, bonus, or shift change may be possible. Always ask for what you desire during negotiations for contract renewal or extension. You will probably get it.

Consider some time off between the end of the current contract and the extension, or renewal, start. If you would like some, arrange it in the contract. Ask the recruiter about paid time off. It usually is not available, but it never hurts to ask.

When taking time off between assignments, renewals, or extensions, be sure to consider your housing. Most companies will not cover housing at the assignment locale for longer than two to three days before and after a contract ends. If you are planning a week off and will be staying at your temporary locale, or just leaving your possessions there, check with a recruiter about the company's policy. Arrangements can usually be made to accommodate the timing. Maybe your belongings could be put in a storage unit, or perhaps, you could pay a portion of the housing cost for that month.

It is possible that time off could be arranged, stated in the contract of course, with a schedule at the facility that will allow for several sequential days off. These days will be related to which days of the week are worked during the last week of current contract and the first week of the new one. Explore all the options. Recruiters are great at working the details out.

> ## Fast facts in a nutshell
>
> - If you are dissatisfied with your current travel staffing company or recruiter, find another one to handle the contract renewal or extension.
> - Contract extension or renewal is a great time to address housing changes, pay increases, time off, and/or a bonus.
> - Clarify housing details when asking for time off between assignments, renewals, and/or extensions.

EXTENSION/RENEWAL NOTIFICATION

By week seven or eight of the assignment, **the nurse manager, or recruiter, may notify you of the availability of a contract renewal or extension.** If not, and you would enjoy either; notify the recruiter and manager ASAP. This allows them time to start planning for the change. It also prevents a search for your replacement. Negotiate, read, and sign the new, or amended, document just as you did the initial travel nurse contract. Note each detail.

Let's discuss one additional tidbit. **Try to wait until at least the seventh or eighth week of an assignment before agreeing in writing to extend or renew.** Occasionally, around this time, things come to light that were not noticed earlier. This is probably because of all the fun you've been having, as well as the newness of the job. It can all produce a "honeymoon" like feeling. Take it from me; I have made the mistake of extending too soon. Work and play while allowing a week or two more to pass, then sign, sign, and sign.

Fast facts in a nutshell: summary

Travel nurse contracts are easily renewed or extended. Negotiations can be performed to allow for changes or additional benefits during this time. Notify the recruiter and nurse manager if you desire an extension or renewal, but wait until week 7 or 8 of the current contract to sign the new agreement. This will give you time and enable you to be certain of the choice.

Chapter 19

Accepting Another Assignment Versus a Permanent Position

INTRODUCTION

Many times, an assignment will not warrant a renewal or an extension. This is not because there have been problems or that you did not like the facility. It is because it is time to move on. It might be that you yearn for a change of location or facility. It could be that you like the facility, but would like to try a different unit. The need for a traveler may no longer exist in the current department. Whatever the reason, the time has come to find a new assignment, search for a permanent position, or possibly return home. Chapter 19 discusses these options and provides guidelines to help determine which step is right for you.

In this chapter, you will learn:

1. How to decide what step to take after each assignment is complete.
2. Where to look for the next travel assignment.

3. What to do when it is time to look for a permanent position and/or return "home."

THE NEXT STEP

Being a travel nurse will be one of the most rewarding experiences of your life. It certainly was for me. I learned so much professionally. I grew enormously on a personal level because of the relationships with those I met while on "the road." I visited locations that I never dreamt I would see.

It is true that adventure alone is a great reason to keep traveling. The friends made along the way are additional rewards. The pay is fabulous and you are constantly learning, while on the job and while exploring your assignment locale. All of these attributes make for a fabulous career. **Job satisfaction is very high among travel nurses** who are in control of their location, facility, and unit, every 13 weeks. A traveler has the ability to change all, or one, of these variables with each new contract.

Because it is great fun and can be lucrative, **it is sometimes hard to know when** to stop. While these things are all fantastic, that same constant change can be taxing over time. Change and distance can be hard on long-term relationships. It is can difficult to advance up the career ladder, if that is a desire. **Travel nurses are truly "travelers,"** and sometimes that is not enough. Therefore, there are several considerations that will help you determine whether to continue traveling or begin looking for a permanent position, either at home or elsewhere.

> ### Fast facts in a nutshell
>
> - Travel nursing is a fantastic, rewarding career.
> - The constant change, distance from loved ones, and temporary staffing situation can become troublesome over a long period of time for some nurses.

The decision to end a traveling career is an individual one. Each person must come to his or her own decision. **Support from friends and family is important.** Making a list of the pros and cons of continued travel is a great way to begin the decision-making process. Be sure to enlist those close to you to help with the process.

> ### Fast facts in a nutshell
>
> Make a decision regarding continued travel only after some consideration and with the support of loved ones.

ACCEPTING ANOTHER ASSIGNMENT

If you desire to continue a traveling career, another assignment is needed. Go back to Part I to review the information about choosing a company, location, facility, and finally, how and when to accept a contract.

Check out a few other travel companies to be sure that you are getting the best care from the one currently used. If you are truly happy with your company and it is a good match, terrific. If not, now is the perfect time to weigh apples to apples and find one that better suits your needs. You can always return to your previous company for another assignment, if desired.

Talk with the other travelers at your facility, as well as any travelers you have met from other hospitals. Find out where they have been and where they would like to go. How did they like the facility, the manager, and the town? What should be seen, what should be skipped? **Learning from others' experiences is a great way to avoid some pitfalls, but always remember to consider the source of the information.**

Other traveling professionals are valuable tools for ideas on where to go, when to be leery, and, sometimes, what to avoid. I have tried to learn from others, as well as from my own mistakes.

It is best to **keep in mind that the traveling medical world is quite small.** Don't burn any bridges you do not have to. A quick example of how close knit this community occurred when I sold a convertible car to a colleague while wrapping up an assignment in Hawaii. About a year later, while on assignment in Alaska, I met a traveler who had just finished an assignment at the same department in the same hospital in which I had worked in Honolulu. While talking about the sites, the food, and the beaches, the traveler mentioned how one of the staff nurses had taken her sightseeing in a white convertible.

Yep, you guessed it. She had ridden in my car. The nurse who purchased it was still employed when this particular traveler was on assignment in Hawaii. She was being a great coworker and took the new trekker sightseeing, in my old car.

The moral of the story is to be nice and stay cordial. **It never hurts to make a good, lasting impression.** I wish I could mention all the times I have experienced, "Oh, I know him!" or "Yeah, I've heard of her." You never know whom you will work with or who will work with you. **Keeping up good contacts also leads to good referrals.**

Fast facts in a nutshell

- Review the information in Part I and compare your current staffing company to a few others before accepting another assignment.
- Other travelers are amazing resources for ideas regarding locations, companies, and facilities.
- Be friendly, positive, professional, proficient, and safe. You may encounter a co-worker, a doctor, or one of their acquaintances on the next assignment.

SEARCHING FOR A PERMANENT POSITION

Travel nursing allows dramatic flexibility throughout your career. You could travel for 6 months, go home for a year, and, then, return to another assignment for 13 weeks. This is only one example showcasing the flexibility of traveling. **The possibilities are endless.** Anything goes, and you can come and go as you please. The schedule is yours to dictate.

If you decide to return "home" for a permanent position or have chosen to accept a permanent position in a different location, **the decision made can never be wrong.** Travel nursing will always be there if you change your mind or just need a little change of latitude. If you do decide to settle down, the experiences of being a traveling professional will always be a part of you.

Fast facts in nutshell

Complete research and consider several options when deciding on a permanent position.

Traveling is an extremely flexible portion of a nursing career that is full of fun, friends, great pay, and adventure.

Fast facts in nutshell

Searching for a permanent position requires as much work as finding an assignment. Research the facility, the unit, and the city. Speak with staff members and anyone local to the area you already know. Weigh the pros and cons, making comparison lists to talk over with friends and family. Choose the position that best suits your needs.

Remember, you are a NURSE, a medical professional whose valuable skills are in demand. The world is your oyster! Good luck and God bless!

Fast facts in a nutshell: summary

Deciding what to do after an assignment is complete is a task that requires much consideration. Listing pros and cons, along with family support makes for a good decision process.

If you decide to continue on the travel nurse adventure, determine the location for another travel assignment using the steps provided in Part I. If a permanent position is desired, complete the proper research and interviews. No matter what arena you work in nursing is an exciting, enriching, rewarding career.

Appendix A

Statement of Health Form Example

SECTION A – MEDICAL RELEASE AUTHORIZATION
(To Be Completed by the Traveler)

I, _____ (client name), do hereby authorize
_____ (physician name) to release any
information acquired during my medical examination to a Travel
Staffing Company.

I also authorize the Travel Staffing Company to release any
information on this statement, relevant to employment, to any of
its client facilities

_____   _____
CLIENT SIGNATURE   DATE

SECTION B – STATEMENT OF PHYSICAL HEALTH
(To Be Completed by the Physician)

I have examined the patient and determined that this person is in good physical and mental health, free of communicable diseases, and able to function and perform all job duties without any physical limitations in his/her profession at full capacity.

Physician Signature   License Number   Date

Physician Name (Please Print)

PHYSICIAN ADDRESS (Please Print):

Street: _____

City: _____ State: _____ Zip: _____

Physician Telephone Number: _____

Appendix B

Do Not Use List

Do Not Use List for Abbreviations, Acronyms, and Symbols

Do Not Use	Potential Problem	Use Instead
U (unit)	Mistaken for "0" (zero), the number "4" (four), or "cc"	Write "unit"
IU (International Unit)	Mistaken for IV (intravenous) or the number 10 (ten)	Write "International Unit"
Q.D., QD, q.d., qd (daily)	Mistaken for each other	
Q.O.D., QOD, q.o.d, clod (every other day)	Period after the Q mistaken for "I" and the "0" mistaken for "I"	Write "daily" Write "every other day"
Trailing zero (X.0 mg)*	Decimal point is missed	Write X mg
Lack of lead in zero .X m		Write O.X mg

(continued)

Do Not Use	Potential Problem	Use Instead
MS	Can mean morphine sulfate or magnesium sulfate	Write "morphine sulfate"
MSO4 and MSO$_4$	Confused with one another	Write "magnesium sulfate"
> (greater than)	Misinterpreted as the number "7" (seven) or the letter "L."	Write "greater than"
< (less than)	Confused with one another	Write "less than"
Abbreviations for drug names	Misinterpreted due to similar abbreviations for multiple drugs	Write drug names in full
Apothecary units	Unfamiliar to many practitioners	Use metric units
	Confused with metric units	
G	Mistaken for the number "2" (two)	Write "at"
cc	Mistaken for U (units) when poorly written	Write "mL" or "ml" or "milliliters" ("mL" is preferred)
pg	Mistaken for mg (milligrams) resulting in one thousandfold	Write "mcg" or "micrograms"

*Exception: A "trailing zero" may be used only where required to demonstrate the level of precision of the value being reported, such as for laboratory results, imaging studies that report sizes of lesions, or catheter tube sizes. It may not be used in medication orders or other medication-related documentation.

Appendix C

Travel Nurse Staffing Companies

This list is arranged in alphabetical order. There are no recommendations made as to which travel staffing company is preferred. Complete your own research to find the company that best suits your personal requirements. This list is in no way a complete compilation of staffing companies, as there are mergers, name changes, and new company start-ups often.

A

Advanced Clinical Employment Staffing, LLC
Voice: 866-864-8620
Web site: www.acesnursetravel.com

Advantage RN
Voice: 866-301-4045
Web site: www.advantagern.com

Alliant Medical Staffing
Voice: 866-868-0469
Web site: www.alliantmedical.com

American Mobile Healthcare
Voice: 800-282-0300
Web site: www.americanmobile.com

American Nursing Services
Voice: 800-444-6877
Web site: www.american-nurse.com

American Traveler Staffing Professionals
Voice: 800-884-8788
Web site: www.americantraveler.com

Aureus Medical Group/Nursing
Voice: 800-856-5457
Web site: www.aureusmedical.com

Axis Healthcare Staffing
Voice: 866-916-AXIS (2947)
Web site: www.axishealthcarestaffing.com

B
Bridge Staffing
Voice: 866-661-7070
Web site: www.bridgestaffing.com

C
Cirrus Medical Staffing
Voice: 800-299-8132
Web site: www.cirrusmedicalstaffing.com

Clinical One
Voice: 800-919-9100
Web site: www.clinicalone.com

CoreMedical Group
Voice: 800-995-2673
Web site: www.coremedicalgroup.com

Critical Options
Voice: 866-274-8677
Web site: www.criticaloptions.com

CrossCountry/TravCorps
Voice: 800 347-2264
Web site: www.crosscountrytravcorps.com

E
Elite Travel Nurse
Voice: 866-448-7444, Voice: 800-894-3107
Web site: www.elitetravelnurse.com

Emerald Health Services
Voice: 800-917-5055
Web site: www.emeraldhs.com

Expedient Medstaff
Voice: 877-EMS-8770
Web site: www.expedientmedstaff.com

F
FASTAFF
Voice: 877-912-9478
Web site: www.fastaff.com

Freedom Healthcare Staffing
Voice: 866-463-0385
Web site: www.freedomhcs.com

H

HEALTHCAREseeker.com
Voice: 888-331-3431
Web site: www.healthcareseeker.com

HRN
Voice: 888-476-9333
Web site: www.hrnservices.com

Health Specialists, Inc.
Voice: 877-NURSEGO
Web site: www.healthspecialists.com

M

Maxim Staffing
Voice: 866-411-2022
Web site: www.maximstaffing.com

Medical Express
Voice: 800-544-7255
Web site: www.medicalexpress.com

Medical Solutions
Voice: 866-633-3548
Web site: www.medicalsolutions.com

Medical Staffing Network, Inc.
Voice: 800-MSN-TEAM
Web site: www.intelistaf.com

MedSource Travelers
Voice: 800-440-1909
Web site: www.medsourcetravelers.com

N

NovaPro Staffing
Voice: 888-668-2779
Web site: www.novaprostaffing.com

NurseChoice
Voice: 866-557-6050
Web site: www.nursechoice.com

Nurse One Staffing
Voice: 800-301-4113
Web site: www.nurseonestaffing.com

Nursing Ventures Inc
Voice: 877-657-6262
Web site: www.nursingventures.com

NursesRx
Voice: 800-735-4774
Web site: www.nursesrx.com

O

Onward Healthcare
Voice: 800-278-0332
Web site: www.onwardhealthcare.com

P

PPR Healthcare
Voice: 866-581-5038
Web site: www.pprhealthcare.com

PRN Health Services
Voice: 888-830-8811
Web site: www.prnhealthservices.com

Q
The Quest Group, Inc
Voice: 866-818-8843
Web site: www.quest-grp.com

Quik Travel Staffing, Inc
Voice: 800-553-2230
Web site: www.qtstaffing.com

S
Sagent Healthstaff
Voice: 877-447-3376
Web site: www.sagenths.com

Soliant Health
Voice: 800-849-5502
Web site: www.soliant.com

Surgical Staff Inc.
Voice: 888-339-9559, Voice: 800-SSI-TRAV
Web site: www.surgicalstaffinc.net

T
TeamStaffRX
Voice: 800-345-9642
Web site: www.teamstaffrx.com

TLC Nursing Services, Inc.
Voice: 800-823-7650
Web site: www.nursestaffing.com

Travel Nurse Solutions
Voice: 888-300-5132
Web site: www.tnsnurse.com

TruStaff
Voice: 877-880-0346
Web site: www.trustafftravelnurses.com

V
Valley Healthcare Systems, Inc
Voice: 800-953-0508
Web site: www2.vhcsystems.com

W
Worldwide Travel Staffing
Voice: 866-633-3700
Web site: www.worldwidetravelstaffing.com

Appendix D

U.S. STATE BOARDS OF NURSING
(On-Line Access)

Alabama Board of Nursing
http://www.abn.state.al.us

Alaska Board of Nursing
http://www.dced.state.ak.us/occ/pnur.htm

Arizona State Board of Nursing
http://www.azbn.gov

Arkansas State Board of Nursing
http://www.arsbn.org

California Board of Registered Nursing
http://www.rn.ca.gov

Colorado Board of Nursing
http://www.dora.state.co.us/nursing

Connecticut Board of Examiners for Nursing
http://www.state.ct.us/dph

Delaware Board of Nursing
http://dpr.delaware.gov/boards/nursing

District of Columbia Board of Nursing
http://hpla.doh.dc.gov/hpla/cwp/view,A,1195,Q,488526,
hplaNav,|30661|,.asp

Florida Board of Nursing
http://www.doh.state.fl.us/mqa

Georgia State Board of Licensed Practical Nurses
http://www.sos.state.ga.us/plb/lpn

Georgia Board of Nursing
http://www.sos.state.ga.us/plb/rn

Guam Board of Nurse Examiners
http://www.dphss.guam.gov

Hawaii Board of Nursing
http://www.hawaii.gov/dcca/areas/pvl/boards/nursing

Idaho Board of Nursing
http://www2.state.id.us/ibn

Illinois Board of Nursing
http://www.idfpr.com/dpr/WHO/nurs.asp

Indiana State Board of Nursing
http://www.in.gov/pla

Iowa Board of Nursing
http://www.iowa.gov/nursing

Kansas State Board of Nursing
http://www.ksbn.org

Kentucky Board of Nursing
http://www.kbn.ky.gov

Louisiana State Board of Practical Nurse Examiners
http://www.lsbpne.com

Louisiana State Board of Nursing
http://www.lsbn.state.la.us

Maine State Board of Nursing
http://www.maine.gov/boardofnursing

Maryland Board of Nursing
http://www.mbon.org

Massachusetts Board of Registration in Nursing
http://www.mass.gov/dpl/boards/rn

Michigan/DCH/Bureau of Health Professions
http://www.michigan.gov/healthlicense

Minnesota Board of Nursing
http://www.nursingboard.state.mn.us

Mississippi Board of Nursing
http://www.msbn.state.ms.us

Missouri State Board of Nursing
http://pr.mo.gov/nursing.asp

Montana State Board of Nursing
http://www.nurse.mt.gov

Nebraska Board of Nursing
http://www.hhs.state.ne.us/crl/nursing/nursingindex.htm

Nevada State Board of Nursing
http://www.nursingboard.state.nv.us

New Hampshire Board of Nursing
http://www.state.nh.us/nursing

New Jersey Board of Nursing
http://www.state.nj.us/lps/ca/medical/nursing.htm

New Mexico Board of Nursing
http://www.bon.state.nm.us

New York State Board of Nursing
http://www.nysed.gov/prof/nurse.htm

North Carolina Board of Nursing
http://www.ncbon.com

North Dakota Board of Nursing
http://www.ndbon.org

Ohio Board of Nursing
http://www.nursing.ohio.gov

Oklahoma Board of Nursing
http://www.youroklahoma.com/nursing

Oregon State Board of Nursing
http://www.osbn.state.or.us

Pennsylvania State Board of Nursing
http://www.dos.state.pa.us/bpoa/cwp/view.asp?a=
1104&q=432869

Rhode Island Board of Nurse Registration and Nursing
Education
http://www.health.ri.gov

South Carolina State Board of Nursing
http://www.llr.state.sc.us/pol/nursing

South Dakota Board of Nursing
http://www.state.sd.us/doh/nursing

Tennessee State Board of Nursing
http://health.state.tn.us/boards/nursing/index.htm

Texas Board of Nursing
http://www.bon.state.tx.us

Utah State Board of Nursing
http://www.dopl.utah.gov/licensing/nursing.html

Vermont State Board of Nursing
http://www.vtprofessionals.org/opr1/nurses

Virgin Islands Board of Nurse Licensure
http://www.vibnl.org

Virginia Board of Nursing
http://www.dhp.virginia.gov/nursing

Washington State Nursing Care Quality Assurance
Commission
https://fortress.wa.gov/doh/hpqa1/hps6/nursing/
default.htm

West Virginia Board of Examiners for Registered
Professional Nurses
http://www.wvrnboard.com

Wisconsin Department of Regulation and Licensing
http://drl.wi.gov

Wyoming State Board of Nursing
http://nursing.state.wy.us

Appendix E

Math Review and Recommended Quick Study Resources

TABLE E.1 Equivalents of Weights and Measures

Liquid Measure	Approximate Apothecary Equivalents	Liquid Measure	Approximate Apothecary Equivalents
Metric		*Weight*	
1000 ml	1 quart	1 Gm	15 grains
500 ml	1 pint	60 mg	1 grain
250 ml	8 fluid ounces	30 mg	$\frac{1}{2}$ grain
30 ml	1 fluid ounce	15 mg	$\frac{1}{4}$ grain
1 Tbsp = 15 ml	4 fluid drams	10 mg	$\frac{1}{6}$ grain
1 Tsp = 5 ml	1¼ fluid drams	0.6 mg	1/100 grain
4 ml	1 fluid dram	0.4 mg	1/150 grain
1 ml	15 minims	0.3 mg	1/200 grain
0.06 ml	1 minim	0.2 mg	1/300 grain

100 micrograms = 1 milligram
1 kilogram = 1000 Gm (2.2 pounds)
1 Gm = 1000mg

CALCULATIONS FOR MCG

$$\text{RATE} = \frac{\text{dose} \times \text{wt} \times 60}{\text{concentration}}$$

or

$$\frac{\text{desired mcg/kg/min} \times \text{pt wt (kg)} \times 60 \text{ min/hr}}{\text{mcg/cc}} = \text{cc/hr}$$

$$\text{DOSE} = \frac{\text{rate} \times \text{concentration}}{60 \times \text{wt}} \text{ or } \frac{\text{cc/hr} \times \text{mcg/cc}}{60 \text{min/hr} \times \text{kg}} = \text{mcg/kg/min}$$

$$\text{CONCENTRATION} = \frac{\text{mg drug} \times 1000 \text{mcg/mg}}{\text{cc diluent}} = \text{mcg/cc}$$

$$\text{DRIP RATE} = \frac{\text{gtt/ml of IV set} \times \text{cc/hr}}{60} = \text{gtt/mnm}$$

$$\text{IV FLOW RATE} = \frac{\text{drops per cc}}{60 \text{ minutes}} \times \frac{\text{amount of fluid per hour}}{1} = \text{gtt/min}$$

REMEMBER: Total Fluid (divided by) Total Number of Hours = Amount
        per hour
        Amount per hour (divided by) 60 minutes = cc per minute
        cc per minute × drops per cc = drops per minute.
        Use a Microdrip system for small amounts of fluid over long
        period of time or per policy.
        Use a Macrodrip system for a large amount of fluid in a short
        time or per policy.

Use the following gtts/ml for the type of tubing you select to use:

Microdrip Tubing = 60 gtts/ml
Macrodrip Tubing = l0 gtts/ml
Blood Tubing = 15 gtts/ml
Intralipid Tubing = 20 gtts/ml

RECOMMENDED QUICK STUDY RESOURCES

Boyer, M.J. (2009). Math for nurses: A pocket guide to dosage calculation and drug preparation (7th Ed). Philadelphia: Wolters Kluwer/Lippincott Williams & Wilkins.

Stassi, M. E., Kaplan, Tiemann, M. A. (2007). Kaplan math for nurses: A pocket skill-builder and reference for dosage calculation. New York: Kaplan Publishing.

Study Guide for PBDS

The Performance Based Development System, or PBDS, is a competency tool created by Dorothy del Bueno. Some of the large hospital systems give this test, however it is not as widely used as some nurses believe. The PBDS is supposed to be given to assess nurses so that an individualized orientation plan can be developed based on the learning needs gleaned from the exam. However, for travel nurses, it is primarily used to determine competency. Failing is uncommon but usually results in termination of the contract.

The majority of the PBDS involves critical thinking skills. Different formats are utilized, such as pen and paper, pictures, and video shorts. This test is not nearly as difficult as it has been rumored to be and there is a good chance you may not encounter it during your travel-nursing career.

A few words of advice: do not forget to include nursing actions that may seem automatic or obvious. If your patient is on IV heparin and begins to vomit blood, stop the heparin. Use your training and common sense. Take your time and re-member to include the obvious answers. Also, ask your travel staffing company if any study guides are available.

Appendix F

Examples of Skills Checklists and Travel Nursing Contracts

1. Example of a Critical Care Skills Checklist from a travel staffing company

This assessment is for determining your experience in the below outlined clinical areas. This checklist will not be used as a determining factor in accepting your application to become an employee.

PROFICIENCY SCALE

1. No Experience   2. Needs Training
3. Able to Perform with Supervision   4. Able to Perform Independently

Proficiency Scale	1	2	3	4
Respiratory				
Administer O2 (NC, Mask)				
Assessment of Breath Sounds				
Assist with Bronchoscopy				
Assist with Chest Tube Insertion				
Assist with Chest Tube Removal				
Assist with Cricothyroid Airway				
Assist with Extubation				
Assist with Intubation				

Proficiency Scale	1	2	3	4
Other				
Advance Directives				
Isolation Techniques				
Post-Anesthesia Care				
Postpartum Care				
Pre-Operative Care/Preparation				
Cardiac				
Assessment of Heart Sounds				

Procedure				Procedure			
Assist with Thoracentesis				Assist with Code			
Draw Blood from Arterial Line				Assist with Open Chest Procedures			
Interpret Arterial Blood Gases				Basic 12-Lead Interpretation			
Perform Arterial Puncture				Cardiac Arrest/CPR			
Pulse Oximetry				Defibrillation/Cardioversion			
Suctioning				Identify Lethal Dysrhythmias			
Troubleshoot Ventilator Problems				Perform 12-Lead EKG			
Use of Assist-Control				Telemetry			
Use of Blow-by				Use of Cardiac Monitors			
Use of CPAP							
Use of ETT CO2 Detectors				Assist with Insertion and Setup:			
Use of Hi-Freq Jet Ventilation				Arterial Lines			
Use of IMV				Central Venous Catheter			
Use of PEEP				Intra-aortic Balloon (IABP)			
Use of Pressure Support				Pericardiocentesis			

(continued)

Proficiency Scale	1	2	3	4
Use of Pressure Ventilators				
Use of Volume Ventilators				
Use of Volume Ambu-bag				
Weaning Patient from Ventilator				
Care of Patient With:				
ARDS				
Assess Resp Complication				
Chest Injury				
ECMO				
Hemo/Pneumo				
Lung Transplant				
Pulmonary Edema				
Tracheostomy				

Proficiency Scale	1	2	3	4
Placement of External Pacemaker				
Pulmonary Artery Catheter				
Obtain/Interpret Hemodynamic Measurements:				
Arterial Pressure (MAP)				
Cardiac Output (Thermodilution)				
Central Venous Pressure				
Intervene PA Catheter Problems				
Obtain ABG				
Obtain Mixed Venous Gases				
PA Pressure				
PCW Pressure				
SVO2				

Emergency Medication Administration:			Care of Patient With:			
Atropine			Acute MI			
Bicarbonate			Aneurysm			
Bretlyium			Automatic Implanted Defibrillator			
Epinephrine			Cardiac Tamponade			
Lidocaine			Cardiogenic Shock			
TPA			Congestive Heart Failure			
			DIC			
Vaso-Active Drips:			Heart Transplant			
Dobutamine			Hypovolemic Shock			
Dopamine			Intra-aortic Balloon Pump (IABP)			
Inocor			Permanent Pacemaker			
Nipride			Pre/Post Cardiac Cath			
Nitroglycerin			Pre/Post Cardiac Surgery			
			Septic Shock			

(continued)

Proficiency Scale	1	2	3	4
Care of Patient With:				
Acute Renal Failure				
Chronic Renal Failure				
Hemodialysis				
Peritoneal Dialysis				
Renal Transplant				
Neurology				
Acute CVA				
Aneurysm Precautions				
Assist with Lumbar Puncture				
Care of Patient With:				
Cerebral Aneurysm				
CNS Infections				

Proficiency Scale	1	2	3	4
Temporary Pacemaker				
Ventricular Assist Device				
Renal				
Acute Renal Failure				
Care of Patient with:				
Chronic Renal Failure				
Hemodialysis				
Peritoneal Dialysis				
Renal Transplant				
Gastrointestinal				
Assessment of Bowel Sounds				
Identification of Abnormalities				

		Item			Item
		Craniotomy			Insert/Maintain Feeding Tubes
		Degeneration Diseases of CNS			Insert/Maintain NG Tubes
		Drug Overdose/DT's			Care of Patient with:
		Epidural Medication Admin			Abdominal Aortic Aneurysm
		Glasgow Coma Scale			Acute Pancreatitis
		Halo Traction/Cervical Tongs			Esophageal Hemorrhage
		Increased ICP			GI Bleed
		Intracranial Pressure Monitoring			Open Abd Wound/Incision
		Neuro Assessment/Vital Signs			Peritoneal Lavage
		Open/Closed Head Injury			
		Seizure Precautions			Other
		Spinal Cord Injury			AIDS
		Use of Rotating Bed			Bone Marrow Transplant
		Use of Stryker Frame			

(continued)

Proficiency Scale	1	2	3	4	Proficiency Scale	1	2	3	4
					Burns				
					Chemotherapy				
					Ketoacidosis				
					Liver Transplant				
					Multiple Trauma				
					Oncology				

The information represented above is true and correct to the best of my knowledge. I also provide authorization to share the above skills checklist with the company's hospital clients.

Signature: _____   Date: _____

Name (printed): _____

2. Example of a travel staffing company Age Specific Competency Form

Place a check in the appropriate column that denotes the level at which you are able to ensure a safe and caring environment for the specific age groups indicated below; able to communicate and instruct patients from the various age groups; and able to evaluate age-appropriate behavior and skills.

PROFICIENCY SCALE
1. No Experience   2. Need Training
3. Able to perform with supervision
4. Able to perform independently

Proficiency Scale	1	2	3	4
Newborn (birth-30 days)				
Infant (30 days-1 yrs)				
Toddler (1-3 yrs)				
Preschooler (3-5 yrs)				
School Age (5-12 yrs)				
Adolescents (12-18 yrs)				
Young Adults (18-39 yrs)				
Middle Adults (39-64 yrs)				
Older Adults (64 yrs +)				

The information represented above is true and correct to the best of my knowledge. I also provide authorization to share the above skills checklist with the company's hospital clients.

Signature: _____ Date: _____

Name (printed): _____

3. Sample Contracts*

Example Contract 1

Example Nursing Company
123 Main Street, Anytown, USA 12345
(555) 555-1212 – www.examplenurses.org

May 31, 2009

Jane Doe
123 Example Sq.
Sometown, USA 54321

Dear Ms. Doe,

Welcome to Example Nursing Company! This letter confirms your assignment with Anytown Regional Hospital in Anytown, USA. The following outlines the details of this assignment:

Unit:	
Shift Assignment:	
Start Date:	
End Date:	
Time Off:	
Base Hourly Rate:	
Overtime Hourly Rate:	
On-Call Hourly Rate:	
Call Back and Holiday Rate:	
Bonus:	
Stipend (per month):	

*These contracts are examples only. No indication of specific guidelines is to be assumed.

Travel Expenses:

You will make arrangements for your travel to Anytown, USA prior to the start of your contract on 00/00/0000. You will receive a one-time travel stipend in the amount of $0.00, received no later than your second paycheck.

Housing:

_____ A private one-bedroom fully furnished apartment with utilities included has been reserved for you at:

_____

Please call _____ (owner) at _____

prior to your arrival on _____ to arrange key pickup.

Example Nursing Company will pay for your housing 48 hours prior to the start of your assignment and 24 hours after the last day of your assignment. If the accommodations are available and you choose to arrive sooner than _____ , or depart later than _____ , you must contact Example Nursing Company prior to signing this agreement to make arrangements for an extended stay.

_____ You will make your own housing arrangements

Local Transportation:

_____ You have declined a rental vehicle

_____ While in Anytown, a rental vehicle has been reserved for you. Please present this reservation code, _____ , along with your driver's license to the Rental Car desk at the Anytown International Airport; DO NOT PRESENT YOUR CREDIT CARD. The Rental Car Agent should use this reservation code to pull up your reservation which will be linked to Example Nursing Company's direct bill account

1) Insurance: You are responsible for insuring the rental vehicle

2) Upgrades: If you choose to upgrade to a different vehicle where the rate is more than the vehicle reserve, any cost difference as a result of the change will be your responsibility. Additional Drivers: If you require additional drivers, they may be added at the counter. Applicable charges will be your responsibility.

3) Fuel Responsibility: It is your responsibility to return the rental vehicle with a full tank of gas. Any additional fuel charges will be your responsibility.

4) Example Nursing Company does not authorize any changes to this reservation without notification and approval.

5) If you choose to turn in your vehicle after _____ , please notify our office prior to signing this agreement to make arrangements for your extended reservation.

Licensure:

_____ You are required to have a current Anytown, USA license for this position prior to 00/00/0000. You will be reimbursed $0.00 for your licensure expense

_____ Licensure is not required for your discipline.

Insurance

_____ You have indicated you wish to decline participating in the Example Nursing Company health care benefit plan. Please complete our waiver and return it to our office.

_____ You have indicated you wish to enroll in the Example Nursing Company health care benefit plan. Please complete our enrollment documents and return them to our office.

Schedule:

You will be scheduled 40 hours per week including holiday weeks. In the event you request time off or volunteer for leave secondary to overstaffing, the leave will be unpaid. In the event you are unable to work scheduled hours to do unforeseen circumstances such as illness or injury, the leave is unpaid and the assignment may be extended to make up the hours missed.

Please call the Anytown office (555-321-4321) and give the administrative coordinator your work schedule as soon are you receive your schedule.

Assignment

If you choose to end the assignment prior to assignment end date, or, if the client terminates your assignment due to your performance, pre-paid travel stipend and local housing stipends will be reimbursed to ENC at a prorated amount. Future reimbursement may be withheld from your earnings.

In the event of an unforeseen, catastrophic circumstance, which renders you unable to complete your assignment, any expenses incurred by Example Nursing Company that cannot be recovered, will be your responsibility. Example Nursing Company will work with you to recover these expenses.

Time Sheets

Timesheets are due in the office by 9 am every Monday morning (Anytown time). Please fax it to 555-555-4321. Your direct deposit will be in your account by noon the following Monday. If your check is mailed, it should be in your mail on the Monday one week after time sheets are due.

Your time sheets must be:
a. Complete
b. Signed by you
c. Signed by your supervisor or his/her designated representative
(Time sheets cannot be forwarded for payment without this signature)

Your paycheck will be directly deposited to the account you indicate on your direct deposit form. If you with to have it mailed, please indicate this on the direct deposit form. The address on your payroll information form is where your paycheck will be mailed until you call and notify Example Nursing Company, otherwise.

Facility and Contact

Anytown Regional Hospital in Anytown, USA
Department Manager's Name: Betty A. Nobody
Department Manager's Phone Number: (555) 456-7890

Emergency and After Hours Contact
If you need assistance after regular business hours please page the on call representative at (555) 098-7654.

Please do not hesitate to contact me at (800) 777-5555, if you have any further questions. Thank you for accepting this assignment at Anytown Regional Hospital.

Sincerely,   Accepted by

_____   _____

Jessica Doe   Example

_____   _____

Date   Typed or printed name

                                    _____

                                    Date

Example Contract 2

CONFIRMATION OF ASSIGNMENT AND TRAVEL AGREEMENT

This is a confidential agreement by and between Nursing Company, Inc. and Jane Doe, who will be assigned by Nursing Company to provide nursing services to Example Memorial Hospital, Anytown, USA. This agreement confirms the complete understanding of the parties with respect to the assignment.

The anticipated dates of service are 0/00/00 through 00/00/00 with possible extension or cancellation. Your compensation for this assignment will be:

$0.00 per hour flat rate
$0.00 for overtime + 8 hours
$0.00 per diem per day
$0.00 per week car allowance
$0.00 housing allowance
per month

$0.00 paid 1st week ending and at the end of your assignment, for a total of $0.00 for travel expenses, (if extended the total travel amount will not change).

$0.00 for on call with 2 hour minimum for all call backs. Call backs will be paid at $0.00 per hour

Other reimbursable expenses: N/A. Must present receipt to be reimbursed.

You are guaranteed payment for Actual Hours Worked for the duration of this assignment; provided, however, this guarantee is not applicable when you take personal time off, vacation, or sick time in any week or if your assignment is terminated either by you voluntarily or pursuant to Additional Terms No. 6 below. Please note, as with any travel assignment, flexibility is essential. Your schedule and duties may need to change according to the needs of the facility during the course of this assignment.

You will be paid overtime according to the labor laws of the state in which you are working.

Your requested days off are: <u>None.</u> You will not be paid hourly wage, per diem, auto, or other expenses for these days. Your assignment will include the following holiday(s): <u>X Day.</u> To receive pay for the above indicated holidays you must comply with the following holiday pay guidelines, if marked with an "X," the following policy(ies) apply to this assignment:

X   If you do not work the holiday, you must work the scheduled day before and the scheduled day after the holiday to qualify for straight time pay up to 40 hours.

N/A   The facility where you have accepted an assignment does not pay for holidays unless you actually work on the holiday during the above-specified hours.

X   The facility where you have accepted an assignment has facility-recognized holidays that are not included in the Nursing Company holiday policy. You are not guaranteed holiday pay for these holidays unless indicated above as a recognized holiday that has been pre-approved by the facility as a recognized holiday for temporary staff.

X   The facility has the option not to schedule you on the holiday and offer hours on another day to guarantee hours for that pay period. If you refuse to work the rescheduled shift, you will not be guaranteed holiday pay and may have per diem, auto, and other expenses pro-rated. Refusing to work the make up shift will be considered a "day off' without pay.

The following policy(ies) also apply to this assignment:

N/A   In addition to the Nursing Company time sheet you must also fax the KRONOS timesheet. If applicable, the additional timesheet must be signed by the facility-designated contact.

X   The pay week for this assignment will be Monday to Sunday.

N/A   At anytime when you do not work a scheduled shift, you must complete a "Guaranteed Hours Verification Form" and have it signed by the authorized facility contact. You will be provided the form at the beginning of your assignment.

N/A The facility where you have accepted this assignment has the right to schedule shifts prior to the end of the assignment or pay period to make up any missed shift.

Additional Terms:

1. This agreement is confidential. Discussion of your compensation package may lead to your termination.

2. Nurse Company will make travel arrangements and provide suitable accommodations for you alone. Any changes in travel arrangements or accommodations will be made solely by Nurse Company. Nurse Company will not be responsible for any changes to travel or accommodations made by you or that have not been approved. You will pay any charges due to damage to the accommodations. Any additional fees or costs associated with housing or travel due to any other person(s) or pet(s) accompanying you on the assignment will be deducted from your paycheck on a weekly basis. By executing this agreement below you are authorizing us to deduct all such amounts from your paycheck.

3. Meals, long-distance phone calls, Internet access, and entertainment are not to be charged to the room and/or apartment. You authorize us to deduct any of these charges from your paycheck if permitted by applicable law.

4. Nurse Company reserves the right to terminate or extend assignments.

5. When signing the rental agreement for the rental car, **DO NOT** accept additional insurance or upgrades. These amounts will be deducted from your pay if you do elect these options, if permitted by applicable law.

6. Per Diems: Please note that if you are receiving a per diem allowance, such an allowance (subject to IRS limits) ordinarily

is not included in your taxable income (Box 1 of your W-2), depending upon, among other factors, the location of your primary residence and length of your scheduled assignment. While Nurse Company monitors the length of your assignment, we ask that you contact us immediately if you change your primary residence during the course of your assignment or if your assignment extends or is scheduled to extend beyond one year. Additionally, this exclusion from taxable income also can have an impact on, among other things, your social security earnings, unemployment compensation, and retirement savings plan contributions (including Nurse Company match). You should consult your accountant or tax advisor regarding your particular situation.

7. If your assignment should terminate due to misconduct, inadequate performance, facility dissatisfaction with your service, and/or your voluntary termination it will be your responsibility to pay for transportation, housing and/or other expenses incurred by Nurse Company after termination of your assignment, which may be deducted from your final check, if permitted by applicable law.

8. You MUST notify Nurse Company immediately when there are changes in your schedule, i.e. personal days not pre-approved or if you call in sick. Nurse Company reserves the right to withhold PER DIEM, AUTO ALLOWANCE, HOUSING ALLOWANCE, and OTHER EXPENSES MADE IN AGREEMENT WITH Nurse Company if you call in sick, elect to take personal days, or if there is no notification of changes in your schedule.

9. There is a 24-hour on-call service to assist you if an EMERGENCY or other urgent situations should arise. The number is 1-800-555-1212.

10. It is your responsibility to fax weekly time sheets to Nurse Company by Monday, 10 am, E.S.T. The time sheet(s) must be verified and signed by the person designated by the facility to

approve time sheet(s). It is your responsibility to verify receipt of your time sheet(s). Failure to comply with this policy may result in delayed payment of your wages.

11. Your employment is temporary and at will. You acknowledge and understand that you are not eligible to participate in <u>Example Memorial Hospital's</u> pension, welfare, or fringe benefit plans or any such plans covering <u>Example Memorial Hospital</u> or its employees, and you shall not seek to participate in any such plans. When your assignment ends, it is your responsibility to report back to Nurse Company for a new assignment. Your failure to do so may affect your eligibility for unemployment benefits.

12. You are required to return this signed agreement prior to the beginning of your assignment. Boarding a flight, accepting a rental car or commencing work at the facility named above constitutes acceptance of the terms of this agreement.

_____   _____

Medical Professional   Jane Doe, Account Manager

_____   _____

Print Name   Date

4. Contract Extension Example

Example Nursing Professionals
2425 South Example Street
Anytown, USA 12345
1.800.888.1234

May 31, 2009
Jane Doe
123 Fake Street
Examplesville, USA 54321

Dear Ms. Doe:

Congratulations on the extension of your assignment! This is a testimony to your professionalism and performance, and we commend you!

***Please sign the EXTENSION TO OUR EXISTING AGREEMENT below, and RETURN THIS DOCUMENT TO ME PROMPTLY VIA FAX.

EXTENSION TO EXISTING AGREEMENT

This agreement serves to document the mutual agreement between the Example Nursing Professionals and myself to extend the length of the term of my original assignment.

The original agreement being referenced is the document entitled "Conditions of Relationship" for the assignment at Example General Hospital in Anytown, USA on 00/00/0000 through the date of 00/00/0000.

This agreement will extend the term of this assignment through the date of 00/00/0000.

STATEMENT OF UNDERSTANDING AND AGREEMENT
I understand that all other terms and conditions set forth in the original agreement remain in force, and my signature below attests to my understanding and agreement to the above-referenced extension.

_____

Jane Doe

_____

Date

_____

I.M. Anexample
Staffing Supervisor
(888) 555-1212
imanexample@examplenursingprofessionals.com

5. Signing Bonus Example

CONFIRMATION OF SIGN ON BONUS AGREEMENT

This is a <u>Confidential</u> Agreement made and entered into by and between Nurse Company and Jane Doe, RN who is in Agreement to provide 00/00/0000 services to 00/00/0000.

This document confirms the complete oral /written understanding of the parties are as follows:

The Sign On Bonus will be for the amount of: $00.00

The Conditions of receiving the Sign On Bonus are as follows:

1. Payment of the Sign On Bonus will be received after 520 hours have been worked on an assignment for Nurse Company.

2. Assignment evaluations from the facility/facilities must be at least 80% and must indicate that the facility /facilities would like you to return.

3. Employee must work a consecutive 520 hours with no time off.

_____   _____

Jane Doe   Date

_____   _____

Nurse Company   Date

Index

Printed in the United States
By Bookmasters